HOT SPOT

How Seattle became *the* place for infectious diseases research

Cover design by Patrick Grandaw

Engel, Mary
Hot Spot: How Seattle became *the* place for infectious diseases research

ISBN 979-8-218-00277-0

Also for sale in ebook format.

1. Medical / Infectious Diseases. 2. Science/ History. 3. Biography & Autobiography/ Medical. 4. Medical/ History

Book design and publishing management by Bryan Tomasovich at The Publishing World

Distributed by Ingram

Printed in the U.S.A.

HOT SPOT

How Seattle became *the* place
for infectious diseases research

MARY ENGEL

HOT SPOT

Author's Note

When Larry Corey approached me about writing a history of the early years of the University of Washington (UW) infectious-diseases program, he explained his motivation for the project this way: "I was trained by the most amazing people in the world."

He wanted the history to explore how Seattle came to develop such a large, comprehensive, and influential program, beginning with good leaders begetting good leaders. And most of all, he wanted to capture the early builders' stories.

That is what this book attempts to do. It covers roughly the period between the arrival of William M.M. Kirby in 1949 to the death of Walter E. Stamm in 2009, with most of the emphasis on fellows from the 1960s, 1970s, and 1980s. For not being able to include all of the remarkable researchers and physician-researchers from this time period, I apologize and hope that I've been able to convey a good sampling of experiences. For those who came later, the work now being done will surely merit its own history.

Because I was still working on this book at the time of the COVID-19 pandemic and because it was hard to ignore, I included a "postscript" on Seattle researchers' early contributions to reining in the pandemic.

Profits from the sale of this book will help fund UW infectious diseases fellowships.

Introduction

Seattle is recognized worldwide as a powerhouse in infectious-diseases (ID) research. How it got there is a storied history, starting with Robert G. Petersdorf, the chair of the University of Washington Department of Medicine who laid its foundation. The first story everyone tells is how he once questioned the demand for the very division he helped build.

"Even with my great personal loyalties to infectious diseases, I cannot conceive of a need for 309 more infectious-diseases experts unless they spend their time culturing each other," he wrote in 1978, referring to the number of ID fellows nationwide scheduled to take the certifying examination that year.[1]

A giant in both ID and in American medical education, Petersdorf was hardly alone in thinking that by the late 1970s, the revolution wrought by better sanitation, vaccines, and antibiotics had lessened the need for his subspecialty. But even as he published the commentary in the *New England Journal of Medicine* arguing for more generalists, a mysterious new illness was beginning to appear.

First reported in 1981, HIV/AIDS would infect millions of men and women worldwide. It and other newly emerging infections, along with reemerging diseases fueled by surging antimicrobial resistance, would prove the continuing need for ID experts. So too would the growing population of people uniquely susceptible to infections, whether due to HIV, cancer treatments that prolonged lives but impaired immunity, or organ transplants that required lifelong immune-suppressing drugs.

Fortunately, the division Petersdorf launched and the physician-researchers trained there were ready to meet the challenge. In fact, Seattle ended up being uniquely well positioned to battle the HIV/AIDS epidemic because of its trailblazing research in three areas.

Sexually transmitted infections (STIs) had not been considered a reputable academic subject of research until an influential UW physician-scientist almost single-handedly made it one, well before HIV hit. Also, before HIV, a UW researcher investigating herpesviruses led clinical trials for the first successful antiviral therapies. And because UW oncologists developed bone marrow transplantation in Seattle, infectious-diseases experts already were learning how to keep patients whose immune systems had been destroyed by treatment from dying of infections.

How did the UW—at the time of Petersdorf's arrival in 1960, still an upstart medical school far from the then-centers of infectious-diseases research—come to be such a leader in the field?

For starters, a trio of stars was already at the UW when or soon after Petersdorf arrived.

William M.M. Kirby came to Seattle in 1949 from Stanford University, recruited by Petersdorf's predecessor to be one of the original members of the Department of Medicine and the first ID specialist in the Pacific Northwest. An expert in tuberculosis and other chest diseases, Kirby was one of the leaders of the antibiotic revolution. He headed the team that invented the Kirby-Bauer antibiotic susceptibility test, which became the standard worldwide for determining which antibiotic to use when treating an infection. It is still in use today.

Kirby's presence helped lure John Sherris, a pioneer in what was then called clinical bacteriology, to the UW from his native England in 1959. Sherris was brought in to run the microbiology laboratory program at the newly opened University of Washington Medical Center. He worked with Kirby and Kirby's fellow, Alfred Bauer, in standardizing the disk diffusion susceptibility test and trained and collaborated with infectious-diseases researchers throughout his long career.

Seymour J. Klebanoff, one of the best white-blood-cell researchers in the world, came to the UW in 1962. He revolutionized science's understanding of the body's infection-fighting immune system. When Kirby decided to step away from administrative duties, Klebanoff became head of the newly combined and renamed Division of Allergy and Infectious Diseases from 1976 to 1994. Like Kirby and Sherris, Klebanoff was known for graciousness and dry, often self-effacing, wit.

And then there was Petersdorf himself.

"He was a builder," said Donald Kaye, a contemporary of Petersdorf's, who was chief of medicine at the Medical College of Pennsylvania around the time Petersdorf was at UW. "He was an unusual person, a force to be reckoned with. Bob Petersdorf built an academic, full-time infectious disease operation in Seattle. The reason he was able to do that was in part because he was Bob Petersdorf."[2]

Petersdorf first came to Seattle to be chief of medicine at Harborview Medical Center, the county-owned, UW-run hospital that was and remains a key clinical teaching site. He had barely arrived when he published a landmark paper on fever of unknown origin with his Yale mentor, Paul Beeson, a legendary physician-scientist who helped shape the field of infectious diseases. Later, Petersdorf became known for his work on endocarditis, begun while on sabbatical with Beeson.

Petersdorf rose to full professor in just two years and became chair of medicine in four. During his tenure as chairman from 1964 to 1979, the UW Department of Medicine overall grew from 69 to 322 full-time faculty members.[3] Among those he lured to Seattle was Beeson, who served as a special advisor to the Puget Sound Veteran's Health Care System and as a source of inspiration to new generations of ID specialists.

During those years, the Department of Medicine ascended the ranks of top medical schools for research funding, solidifying a position in the top 10 along with Harvard, New York, Duke, Columbia, Stanford, UC San Francisco, and Johns Hopkins.

Within the larger UW department, the ID division flourished, with Petersdorf's presence helping to attract stellar faculty, who in turn drew class after class of promising fellows. These fellows went on to build their own programs at the UW and at academic and government centers across the country and the world.

Marvin Turck arrived in 1960 when Petersdorf asked the Public Health Service's Epidemic Intelligence Service (EIS) for an officer to investigate an outbreak of Gram-negative infections at Harborview. According to Turck, Petersdorf was expecting someone more experienced, but Turck impressed his mentor enough to be asked to join the UW faculty in 1964, after completing his residency in Chicago.[4] His research focused primarily on urinary tract infections (UTIs), and he worked with Kirby and Sherris to expand the Kirby-Bauer technique to test Gram-negative bacteria.

But what Turck did best and enjoyed the most was the clinical practice and teaching of medicine. He won the Department of Medicine teaching award so many times that the department finally renamed it the Marvin Turck Outstanding Teaching Award in his honor. He edited the influential *Journal of Infectious Diseases* for 13 years, becoming a mentor to junior faculty members at the UW and across the country, many of whom he invited to review articles.

The Seattle model

Turck's first fellow was a young Canadian physician intrigued by infectious diseases and drawn to the UW by Petersdorf's reputation. Allan Ronald trained under Turck from 1965 to 1967 and stayed an extra year to work with Sherris. Ronald returned home to Winnipeg to build Canada's first infectious-diseases research program—the first of many started by UW fellows. Later, he began a partnership in Nairobi that became one of the longest-running research collaborations in Africa as well as one of the first to incorporate and expand in-country expertise in infectious diseases. Of the more than 30 fellows and house staff that Turck personally mentored, Ronald held a special place in his memory.

So did King Holmes, Turck's first chief resident.

Holmes arrived in Seattle in 1968 with medical degree from Cornell and a PhD in microbiology from the University of Hawaii. In a UW career spanning the next five decades, he became a key figure in the division's history and in infectious-diseases research worldwide.

Continuing a line of investigation that he had begun while serving in the West Pacific for the Navy, Holmes made the study of

STIs not just a respectable focus of academic research but essential for dealing with the AIDS pandemic to come. Working with his first three research fellows—Paul Wiesner, H. Hunter Handsfield, and James Harnisch—he forged a partnership between the UW and the county public health department so that the department had access to the analytic capacity of the university, and university researchers had access to the patients and data accrued in the STI clinic. The "Seattle model" of academic-public health partnership soon became the national standard for sexually transmitted disease (STD) prevention, treatment, and research.

If Petersdorf excelled at building and leading and Turck's forte was the clinical practice and teaching of medicine, Holmes's superpower was a big-picture mind that could make connections no one else saw—whether evaluating the data in a single research project, merging university and county-health interests, or broadening the field of infectious diseases itself. Infectious diseases weren't over just because fewer people were showing up in hospitals near death. Infections could be asymptomatic in one person and damaging in another or driven underground in marginalized and stigmatized populations. To stop them would require not just medical but behavioral and public-health interventions, not just going from bench to bedside but from bench to bedside to communities on a national and international scale.

Holmes joined Ronald in the Nairobi program and eventually formed research partnerships throughout Africa, Southeast Asia, South America, the Caribbean, and the Western Pacific. His work on AIDS and in STIs internationally helped shape the emerging field of global health, and later in his career he became the founding director of a new UW Department of Global Health.

One reason that UW's reach is so great is that good leaders beget good leaders.

"It was Petersdorf who recruited Marvin, who in turn recruited King and others," said Edward W. "Ned" Hook III, who had been chief resident under Turck in 1979 and then a senior ID fellow under Holmes from 1980 to 1983. "Petersdorf was key to the whole thing. He was larger than life."[5]

They all were. This larger-than-lifeness was expressed in their work and also in their personalities.

Petersdorf was an iconoclast with a sharp wit and an unflappable calm. Although he could be gruff and a little scary to medical students and fellows, he had a keen eye for talent.

Turck's clinical skills were so prodigious that he was universally acclaimed as the person UW medicine residents and ID fellows most wished could take their board exams for them. He also always had a joke or three at the ready, having put himself through college working from time to time as a stand-up comedian.

And Holmes had an agile and curious mind, whether for research or in conversation, and a social intelligence that could put anyone, from any culture, at ease.

Other influential early leaders included Harry Beaty, an expert in bacterial meningitis, who put himself through college and medical school at the UW, then did his residency there and trained with Petersdorf as an ID fellow in 1961. After a stint at the National Institutes of Health (NIH), Beaty returned at Petersdorf's invitation to join the faculty in 1965 and took over from Turck as head of infectious diseases at Harborview. One of Beaty's most prominent fellows was George Counts, who also arrived at the UW in 1965 after being recruited by Turck. The son of Oklahoma sharecroppers, Counts would become known not just for his patient care, teaching, and research—on hospital-acquired infections and later on HIV—but as an extraordinary mentor for minority physician-researchers.

It wasn't just these early leaders who made Seattle a force in infectious diseases. It was the fellows they attracted and adopted for life, the fertile exchange of ideas they fostered, and the sense of fellowship that lasted long after the formal training period ended. Fellows learned not just from their mentors but from each other and made contacts that would influence their careers for years to come.

Field of giants

Holmes trained more than 150 of them himself, starting with Paul Wiesner, who, after his fellowship ended, would go on to become the director of the Division of Sexually Transmitted Diseases at the Center for Disease Control[6] in Atlanta. Wiesner became the first of many Holmes fellows to hold influential national and international positions in the field.

Hunter Handsfield and James Harnisch began their fellowships just after Wiesner. Within three years, these early fellows, led by Holmes, made dramatic advances in the clinical science of gonorrhea. Handsfield worked out the until-then unrecognized role and surprising frequency of asymptomatic gonorrhea in men. Wiesner and Harnisch conducted the first comprehensive studies of the clinical manifestations and epidemiology of gonorrhea in men who have sex with men. Wiesner and Handsfield, following up on earlier work by Holmes, Beaty, and Counts, conducted the first large-scale studies of the clinical manifestations and treatment of disseminated gonococcal infection. All of them designed and conducted research into gonorrhea treatment at a time when antibiotic resistance was just being recognized as a disturbing national trend.

Another early fellow, David A. Eschenbach, became the nation's first obstetrician-gynecologist to be formally trained in infectious diseases and, with his mentor, began groundbreaking studies in the clinical aspects and epidemiology of pelvic inflammatory disease (PID).

Handsfield in later years became director of Seattle–King County Public Health's Sexually Transmitted Disease Control Program, which in turn became the widely copied "Seattle model" for public health department–academic center collaboration. Harnisch, who went on to train in dermatology, became a nationally recognized expert on Hansen's disease, or leprosy, and opened a federally funded leprosy clinic in Seattle. Eschenbach continued to research the clinical aspects of PID and other STD problems in women. He became the chair of UW's Department of Obstetrics and Gynecology and cofounded the Infectious Diseases Society for Obstetrics and Gynecology.

And those were just King's first fellows.

Another particularly influential trio arrived in the early to mid-1970s, associated, as Turck had been, with the EIS.

Walter E. Stamm first came to the UW as Turck's chief resident and returned after a stint at the EIS. He fused Turck's research into UTIs with King's research in STDs. Stamm began investigating chlamydia, then newly recognized as the most common bacterial STD. His research on chlamydia and its main complication, PID—one of the main causes of female infertility—led to chlamydia control programs nationwide that dramatically reduced infertility, ectopic pregnancies, and deaths. A leader of uncommon grace, Stamm followed Klebanoff as head of the Division of Allergy and Infectious Diseases from 1994 to 2007. He stepped down after being diagnosed with terminal metastatic melanoma, a loss that, more than a decade on, still made those who knew him tear up.

Joel Meyers came to investigate a hepatitis outbreak during the early years of bone marrow transplantation and stayed to make Seattle a center of research into infections unique to people with compromised immune systems. Despite a life cut short by colon cancer at age 46, Meyers's legacy continues in the research area he pioneered and in the graduates of the Joel Meyers Endowment Scholarship established in his name.

Larry Corey sealed his reputation as a force in infectious diseases early on by leading clinical trials on the world's first antiviral therapy, acyclovir, to control and suppress genital herpes. These early studies paved the way for antiviral therapies for HIV, as well as for hepatitis B and C. Then Corey turned to the biggest challenge of all—working to develop a preventive vaccine against HIV.

"Here were these giants in the field, or they were becoming giants," said Thomas Quinn, recalling arriving at the UW as a Holmes fellow in 1979 and meeting that first week with Holmes, Handsfield, Stamm, Corey, and Harnisch. Quinn went on to be the chief of the NIH's international HIV/STD section and founding director of Johns Hopkins University Center for Global Health.

To understand how thoroughly Holmes and his fellows dominated STD research, consider that in 1983, the American Sexually Transmitted Diseases Association honored King with its preeminent recognition, the Thomas Parran Award (now the Distinguished Career Award). Since then, 14 of his fellows have received the lifetime award.[7] More than a dozen have received the association's Achievement Award recognizing an outstanding body of work at midcareer.

The field expands

The early classes of fellows, along with the early faculty, were mostly men whose introduction to infectious-diseases research often began in the military or in the then-male-dominated EIS. But that would change under Holmes and his fellows. More than half of Holmes's trainees were women.

Sheila Lukehart was one of the first, arriving in 1979 to continue the work on syphilis she had begun as a graduate student at the University of California Los Angeles. She became universally acknowledged as the world's top expert in the biology and immunology of syphilis. She also went on to become the UW School of Medicine's associate dean for research and graduate education and to direct the STD and AIDS training grant started by King more than 40 years ago.

"King fostered women long before it became fashionable to do so," said Ann Collier, a 1982 fellow. "He is incredibly supportive if you are hardworking and have ideas. Now our division has just incredible women. That was King and his disciples."[8]

Collier worked with two of those disciples. She started out in the very early days of the HIV epidemic training under Handsfield, who recruited her. She became the director of the AIDS Clinical Trials Unit under Corey, who was the unit's principal investigator as well as chair of the nationwide AIDS Clinical Trials Group (ACTG). Collier cofounded the Madison Clinic, one of the first clinics in the country devoted entirely to AIDS patients.

Judith Wasserheit was another 1982 fellow, training under Holmes and also with David Eschenbach. She became the founding chief of the NIH's Sexually Transmitted Disease Research Branch, then led the US Centers for Disease Control's (CDC's) Division of STD/HIV Prevention. After her stints at the NIH and the CDC, she returned to the UW, first as director of Corey's HIV Vaccine Trials Network, then succeeded Holmes as chair of the UW Department of Global Health.

Anna Wald worked first with Collier, then in 1991 became a senior fellow under Corey. She followed him as director of the UW Virology Research Clinic and in 2017 became the first woman to head the Division of Allergy and Infectious Diseases.

Part of what drew Jeanne Marrazzo, who began her fellowship a year after Wald and trained under Handsfield, was the sheer number of, at that point, midcareer but advancing women faculty. At the time, she said, "It was incredibly unusual."[9] As a UW faculty member, Marrazzo codirected the STD training grant with Lukehart and did groundbreaking work on the vaginal microbiome with colleague David Fredricks. She left the UW in 2016 to become director of the infectious-diseases division at the University of Alabama—succeeding Ned Hook, who had set up the "Seattle model" first in Baltimore and then in Birmingham.

The Seattle draw

Ask any former fellow what stood out about their fellowship years in Seattle, and they say similar things: the gifted mentors and the commitment to training; an environment that fostered ambitious research without ever losing its emphasis on patient care; the chance to do translational work that went from bench to bedside to community; the big ambition and yet the insistence on collaborative research—not just among themselves but integrating basic science with epidemiology and public health, behavioral research and implementation science, as well as other specialties like dermatology, obstetrics-gynecology, and neurology.

"There was a feeling that whatever came along, we could research it, adapt to it clinically, teach it," said Wesley Van Voorhis, a 1986 fellow under Klebanoff who headed the division from 2007 to 2017.[10]

The UW's abundance of affiliated clinical sites allowed room for an unusually large concentration of ID specialists to set up laboratories and research groups. Petersdorf first landed at Harborview, and the county-owned hospital remained a favorite spot for him to station promising young physician-researchers even after he ascended to chairmanship of the full department. The University of Washington Medical Center opened in 1959—Kirby and Sherris were based there—but the medical school had relationships with a variety of other clinical teaching sites, including, over the years, the US Public Health Service Hospital, the Seattle Veterans Affairs (VA) Medical Center, Seattle Children's Hospital and Fred Hutchinson Cancer Research Center (Fred Hutch). Each offered a specific niche. Harborview had the very serious diseases seen in county hospitals. Until the Public Health Hospital was decommissioned and closed, it offered abundant research space. Fred Hutch focused on immune-compromised patients.

But always, the ethos called for partnerships, not silos. There were egos, sure, but Seattle—the West Coast in general—was largely seen as collaborative and collegial. "We have just amazing relationships that wouldn't happen on the East Coast," Van Voorhis said.

Holmes, for example, was always "King," where it would have been unheard of on the East Coast for a fellow to be on first-name basis with a mentor. (Petersdorf, despite his own preference for the West

Coast, was always "Dr. Petersdorf.") Holmes's research on STIs may well have taken root here in part because the liberal West Coast was more open not only to different views of sexuality but to the broad-minded thinking and collaboration he favored.

Petersdorf left the UW in 1979, but Seattle would eventually draw him back. He moved to Boston for a brief stint as president of the Brigham and Women's Hospital, then—missing both the West Coast and academic medicine[11]—he became vice chancellor for health sciences and dean of the School of Medicine at the University of California, San Diego, from 1981 to 1986. From there he served as the influential president of the Association of American Medical Colleges, a position he held until 1994 and one of many that showcased his natural strength as a leader. He edited one of medicine's leading textbooks and was a policy adviser to federal agencies.

In 1995, he returned to Seattle where, as Paul Beeson had done before him, he served as an adviser at the Seattle VA Medical Center and to the dean of the UW medical school as well as a distinguished professor of medicine.

Ann Collier, immersed in HIV/AIDS work, met him for the first time then. Referring to his long-ago commentary on the declining need for infectious-diseases researchers, Petersdorf told her, "You made me eat my words."[12]

What follows is a history of these early leaders of the UW infectious-diseases division and their influence on Seattle, the nation, and the world.

1

The

Builder

Robert G. Petersdorf met the man who would become his lifelong mentor and friend one March evening in 1952 over a dinner of kale—always kale—in the New Haven Hospital cafeteria.[13] It was rare enough for any Yale School of Medicine faculty member to frequent the hospital's spartan dining room. Even more unheard of, the man who sat down next to the fourth-year medical student and asked about his future plans was Yale's newly arrived chair of medicine, Paul Beeson.

Years later, when Petersdorf had gone on to become a legend in medicine himself, he would also surprise medical students, house staff, and junior faculty by showing interest in them, albeit a gruffer version than the ever-courtly Beeson's. And like Beeson, he had a gift for spotting—and promoting—talent.

Petersdorf even back then was hard to miss. His class standing, work ethic, and assurance during grand rounds already had earned him a prestigious Yale internship.

He was born in Berlin on February 14, 1926, the first of two sons to Hans Petersdorf, a retail businessman, and Sonja, a fashion designer. He was two when the family moved to the United States, first to New York, where they stayed long enough for the young Petersdorf to become a Giants fan, then to California. Graduating from high school in Los Angeles as World War II raged, he finished one year at

1

the University of Wisconsin before serving in the US Army Air Force from 1944 to 1946.

Petersdorf credited his interest in medicine—and infectious diseases—to being given the job of presenting venereal-disease lectures and movies to incoming recruits at Fort Bragg.[14] Upon leaving the service, he completed his bachelor's degree at Brown University in 1948 and entered medical school at Yale. Meeting Paul Beeson reinforced his decision.

Beeson's life spanned 20th century medicine. He grew up in Anchorage, Alaska, the son of a general practitioner who worked for the Alaska Railroad. In 1921, when Beeson was 12 years old, his father traveled more than 800 miles by train and then dog sled to deliver antitoxin to a suspected diphtheria patient in Nome, a feat still commemorated today by the annual Iditarod Trail Sled Dog Race. Beeson would recount the saga to generations of physician trainees.

After completing his undergraduate degree at the University of Washington, Beeson entered medical school at McGill University in Montreal and did his internship at the University of Pennsylvania. He briefly joined his older brother and father—by then in Ohio— in private practice, but a desire to gain more experience in surgery and obstetrics led him to seek additional training in New York. There, after a chance encounter with an old friend from his undergraduate years, he applied for a residency at the Rockefeller Institute for Medical Research.

It was 1937, before the post-war boom of research money and laboratories, and the institute, funded by private philanthropy, was then unique in the United States for its focus on research. Assigned to the pneumonia service, Beeson instantly saw the benefit of combining clinical and laboratory investigation. Before the introduction of antibiotics, pneumonia killed more than 50,000 Americans a year. But researchers were learning to identify pneumococcus species and treat them with type-specific antiserum, the first effective management of lobar pneumonia. This breakthrough was soon replaced by an even more effective one, the antibacterial sulfa drugs.

Medicine was entering an era of rapid change, and Beeson was excited to be on the front lines. Later, Petersdorf would recall his mentor advising him over that very first (kale) dinner that the secret to success in academic medicine was "to get one's hands dirty in the lab."[15]

If his time at Rockefeller ignited his interest in research, Beeson's next position—as chief resident to Soma Weiss at Boston's Peter Bent Brigham Hospital—lit a passion for teaching. Physicians from all over Boston would go to hear Weiss give rounds. The chief of medicine made a point of including patients in his bedside instruction, treating them with a compassion that reminded Beeson of his father.

After a war-time stint in England working for the American Red Cross-Harvard Field Hospital Unit, Beeson put Weiss's lessons into practice at the Emory School of Medicine in Atlanta, where he served as an inspiring chief of medicine. His leadership style, including the passion for teaching and compassion for patients carried on from Weiss, in turn made a lasting impression on Petersdorf, starting with the first of many dinners in that spare hospital dining room.

"We made friendships that have endured"

Throughout his Yale internship and a year of residency, Petersdorf was "dazzled by pearls" dropped by Beeson and by Ivan Bennett, Beeson's former chief resident at Grady Hospital in Atlanta, who followed him to Yale as a fellow. Beeson was hired with the mandate to expand the department and propel it to the ranks of Harvard, Johns Hopkins, and Columbia.[16] Petersdorf witnessed the beginning of that transformation.

"It was an exciting time," Petersdorf later wrote. "We opened up a new hospital unit, we worked hard, including in our workload a great deal of lab work, and we made friendships that have endured. ... Beeson's service provided an environment where everyone thrived."[17]

Beeson was a hero to the house staff not just for his wisdom but for his political courage. More than 40 years later, Petersdorf recalled how, during the red-baiting McCarthy era, Beeson took up the cause of a resident who had been accused of being a communist and called to testify before a congressional committee. The chairman of the Yale-New Haven Hospital Board of Trustees wanted to fire the resident on the spot. Beeson interceded, allowing him to finish the year and then getting him a job with an old friend who was chairman of medicine in Salt Lake City.[18]

After Petersdorf completed his internship and a year of residency in New Haven—six years total, counting medical school—Beeson encouraged him to go somewhere other than Yale for further training. On Beeson's recommendation, Petersdorf got a coveted senior assistant residency at one of Beeson's old stomping grounds, the Brigham Hospital in Boston. From there, he went to Johns Hopkins in Baltimore in the summer of 1955, where Ivan Bennett had taken a position.

Johns Hopkins had a deep tradition of research into infectious diseases before ID was considered a subspecialty, dating back to the work of internist William Osler—one of the medical school's founders in the late 1880s and the author of an influential textbook. Bennett came on board to lead the school's first administratively distinguished Division of Allergy and Infectious Diseases. His research focused on how infectious agents, primarily Gram-negative organisms, interact with host defense systems to produce fever and septic shock.

For Petersdorf, the highlight of his time at Hopkins was the arrival of a new fellow the following year, Edward W. Hook Jr., who would become a lifelong collaborator and friend. Ed Hook hailed from South Carolina by way of Emory University School of Medicine. Though a year behind Petersdorf in the fellowship, Hook had already completed two years in a bacteriology fellowship at Emory and four years of house-staff training at the University of Minnesota and at Grady Hospital in Atlanta. Hook and Petersdorf collaborated on studies on the efficacy of antibiotics in Gram-negative infections.

They played as hard as they worked, taking turns with other house staff hosting legendary parties, the most infamous being those Hook organized. (Bennett was the only faculty member with the courage to attend.) More importantly, in Petersdorf's eyes, Hook knew how to drive—and taught Petersdorf.

"This task was not devoid of risk," Petersdorf would later write. "However, except for an unexpected trip across a neighbor's front lawn, we both survived it."[19]

Still, despite Beeson's earlier advice about the importance of getting his hands dirty in the laboratory, Petersdorf found himself missing clinical medicine. His first few months in the lab were discouraging. He was seriously considering going into practice with Kaiser-Permanente when Beeson came to the rescue and offered him the chief residency at Yale from 1957 to 1958.

"It was that single action that hardened my resolve to stay in academic medicine," Petersdorf later wrote, "a decision I have never regretted."[20]

Fever of unexplained origin

When Petersdorf arrived to begin his chief residency in June 1957, Beeson was across the country tending to an ailing parent.

"It is going to be your service anyway," he wrote in a note left for Petersdorf, "and you might as well start running it now."[21]

Thus began a tradition carried down through Petersdorf and those he trained of hiring capable people and then giving them full responsibility to do their job. Petersdorf later joked that his career peaked during that "heady experience" as Beeson's chief resident.

But there also was time together to learn from his mentor. Petersdorf described how he would do the preliminary history and physicals for patients referred to Beeson, then watch with admiration as his mentor took the time to deal with them "as people rather than as diseases." That lesson never left him.

Beeson also drew him back into research doing influential work on fever. Beeson's earlier studies, some of them undertaken with Bennett, had upended the notion that fever is caused by a foreign organism, as had been the theory, arguing that it was instead the bodily response to an attack. He was the first to identify proteins in white blood cells now recognized as cytokines, which play a role in the body's response to infections. When Petersdorf became chief resident, Beeson asked him to begin working out the details for a paper describing a prospective study of 100 patients with an illness of more than three weeks' duration and episodic fever, who remained undiagnosed after one week in the hospital.

The paper they coauthored, "Fever of Unexplained Origin," was considered a landmark when published in the journal *Medicine* in 1961 and became one of the most frequently cited articles in medical literature.[22] Its findings grouped fevers into various categories—due to infections, malignancies, inflammatory or rheumatological diseases, miscellaneous, and undiagnosed—by percentages that have remained surprisingly consistent through the decades, with some variation in tropical and subtropical settings. Knowing the most common causes of fever and their probabilities gave physicians diagnostic guidelines in the days before high-tech scans and genetic testing.

(The paper included a tongue-in-cheek footnote on "Sutton's Law," named after the bank robber Willie Sutton who, when arrested, was asked by a reporter, "Why do you always rob banks?" and allegedly replied, "Why, that's where the money is." The footnote credited Dr. William Dock for first applying this term to medicine on teaching rounds attended by Beeson and Petersdorf.)

As satisfying as his chief residency had been, Petersdorf declined Beeson's offer to stay on as a faculty member at Yale. Beeson was, after all, leaving that year on a sabbatical. And besides, Ivan Bennett offered him more money—$8,000 a year—to go back to Hopkins' new infectious-diseases division.

So Petersdorf rejoined his friend Ed Hook at Hopkins, until Hook left in 1959 to become head of the Division of Infectious Diseases at Cornell. (An internationally recognized expert in the field, Hook went on to help found the Infectious Diseases Society of America in 1963 and would later serve as its president.) Petersdorf also stayed in close touch with Beeson, tied by friendship, joint research interests, and regular attendance at an informal gathering of infectious-diseases researchers dubbed the Interplanetary Society but more widely known as the Pus Club.[23]

Before the Infectious Diseases Society of America, there was the Pus Club. It was formed around 1940 by Beeson and his close friends Walsh McDermott, who was based at Cornell and New York Hospital, and W. Barry Wood, who spent most of his career at Johns Hopkins.[24] All three were renowned for their leadership skills, their collegiality, and their wide-ranging interests. All became legends in the infectious-diseases field. The Pus Club met once or twice a year and included each scientist's research group and, eventually, their mentees too. Petersdorf was a regular.

In 1960, Petersdorf received an intriguing invitation from clear across the country. Robert H. Williams, the founding chairman of the Department of Medicine at the still-young University of Washington School of Medicine in Seattle, offered him a position as an associate professor and as chief of medicine at Harborview Medical Center, the county-owned, UW-operated hospital and clinical teaching site.

Petersdorf once again turned to Beeson for advice. The UW was, after all, his mentor's undergraduate alma mater and Seattle his old stomping grounds.

"He told me then," Petersdorf wrote, "that the University of Washington was a very young school that was doing almost everything right and that I would be privileged to be part of that building process."

And, Petersdorf added, "He was absolutely right."[25]

It was in Seattle that Petersdorf would reveal his strength as a builder.

The giant in residence: William M.M. Kirby

An endocrinologist renowned for his diabetes research, Robert H. Williams had come to the newly created medical school from Harvard in 1948. He had quickly set about filling his new department with rising stars from around the country.

One of the first, lured from Stanford in 1949 to become the first infectious-diseases specialist in the Pacific Northwest,[26] was William Murray Maurice Kirby.

It was the University of Washington's fortune that Kirby chose medicine over music. Born in Springfield, South Dakota, in 1914, he and his identical twin, Charles, were gifted at both violin and piano, earning summer income playing as a duo on Missouri River cruises.[27] They both considered attending the Oberlin Conservatory of Music but opted instead for premed at Trinity College in Connecticut. From there, they went to Cornell University Medical College, graduating in 1940 and continuing on for a year of internship.

The twins looked so alike it could be unsettling. According to Bill Kirby's daughter, Barbara, Bill Kirby recounted once walking down a hallway calling out "Hello, Charles" before crashing into a mirror. But, although close, the two had very different personalities, which Bill Kirby's children describe as matching the coast where each wound up. (According to family lore, someone sat them down at the end of their internship and said, enough is enough, you need to go your separate ways.)

Charles Kirby headed east, to the University of Pennsylvania, where he became a high-powered cardiothoracic surgeon and professor of surgery, coauthoring an influential manual on chest surgery. His great ambition had been to perfect an implantable artificial heart, a model of which he kept in a desk drawer. But in 1963, at age 49, he died of a heart attack—a loss felt keenly by his surviving twin.

Bill Kirby had headed west to Stanford to be assistant and then chief resident in medicine at Stanford University Hospital. His work ethic and intellectual curiosity equaled his brother's but was balanced by what everyone who met him described as sheer niceness. At Stanford and throughout his career, he combined a passion for patient care and a drive for research with such civility, modesty, and good humor that his three children, all of whom grew up to become physicians, learned about his most influential research from others. Until the day he died, he was a man who loved his work, and showed it.

In the days before infectious-diseases fellowships, Kirby made time during his Stanford residency to do research on the side, focusing on the use of sulfonamides, the forerunners of the antibiotic revolution, in the lab of Dr. Lowell Rantz. There he also met Georgiana Dole, known as Jinx, a bacteriologist who, in 1938, had been one of five women graduating from Stanford in that field. Her name appears on some of the papers Kirby produced over those years. A romance bloomed, but Dole wanted time to think about it and headed to Boston to work for a year in the laboratory of Harvard Medical School's Maxwell Finland, Rantz's mentor and a major force in infectious-diseases research. Before the year was up, her family got a letter announcing, "I'm going back to San Francisco to marry Bill."

By then, Kirby was heading into the US Army and, convinced he would be sent overseas, had set about learning German. Instead, he, like Petersdorf, stayed at Fort Bragg, where he served as a captain and a medic from 1944 to 1947 and took part in some of the earliest studies of what would become the wonder drug of the 20th century—penicillin. Jinx Kirby worked in the bacteriology lab there as well.

The antibacterial effects of the *Penicillium* mold had been discovered and named by the Scottish microbiologist Alexander Fleming at London University in 1928. But it wasn't until World War II that researchers across the country and the world worked together in a government-funded program to develop and mass-produce the drug, driven by the urgent need to treat soldiers wounded on battlefields and to get soldiers infected in brothels back out onto the battlegrounds.

Along with recognition of the drug's miraculous healing powers came the first signs of antimicrobial resistance. Having earlier written on resistance to sulfa drugs, Kirby in 1945 published his discovery of staphylococcal penicillinase, a penicillin inactivator extracted from resistant staphylococci.[28]

Following his Army stint, Kirby, like Beeson, put in a short stay as a visiting investigator at the Rockefeller Institute for Medical Research. He also began developing expertise in infectious chest diseases.

Driving back across the country to the San Francisco Bay Area, he and Jinx stopped in Denver to spend several months at the National Jewish Medical and Research Center, then called the National Jewish Hospital for Consumptives and still among the best worldwide for research and treatment of tuberculosis (TB). Colorado had once been known as the world's sanitorium because of the belief that the disease could be cured by high altitude, abundant sunshine, and fresh air. By the 1940s and into the late 1950s, researchers began treating TB first with streptomycin and then combinations of drugs.

Kirby was back at Stanford as an instructor in medicine when Williams recruited him to the UW.

Part of the attraction to the start-up medical school in the Pacific Northwest may have been that it meant a homecoming for Jinx, by then pregnant with their first child. Jinx had grown up in Hoquiam, Washington, after her father, a cousin of the Hawaiian Dole pineapple clan, settled in the Olympic Peninsula to run the Aloha Mill & Lumber Company. After moving to Seattle, the Kirbys had three children in quick succession, each of whom, infused with their father's enthusiasm for his work, grew up to become physicians.

"He loved it—that's why we all went into medicine," said Barbara Kirby, the eldest, who, like her father, specialized in infectious diseases. "There wasn't any pressure. We saw a very happy father and a very happy life."

Richard Kirby, the youngest, who became an orthopedic surgeon, recalled how their father approached medicine like "a great mystery to be solved," describing cases in detail and challenging his children to reach a diagnosis.

"At the dinner table, he would begin, 'I saw the most interesting patient,'" Richard Kirby said. "We would always hang on to every word." Richard's future wife, Betsy, whom he started dating when they were 13, was less fond of certain topics and at some point, asked, "Can we please not discuss pus at the dinner table?"

Kirby's children were less aware of their father's steely side, exhibited in a campaign to convince Seattle health authorities to abandon local TB sanatoriums once combination drug treatment had been found effective. John Sherris, who came to UW from England in 1959 to join and eventually chair its Department of Microbiology, recalled how Kirby "had big fights with the authorities over this."

"He won pretty quickly," Sherris said. "He could be a tiger if he disapproved of something. You'd never know it from talking to him. You'd see the ultimate gentleman, so easy to get along with. But there was iron in his soul."[29]

A legendary microbiologist: John Sherris

Kirby had been one of the draws to Seattle for Sherris.

"Dr. Kirby was a hero of mine," he said. "He was just simply a superb and very experienced physician with microbiological knowledge and able to work in both microbiology and medicine."[30]

Sherris also straddled both worlds. Born in 1921, he was the son of a small-town general practitioner. In the days before many people had telephones, his father would conduct late-night consultations from Sherris's bedroom window overlooking the front porch. That was his introduction to medicine.

In medical school during World War II, he met his future wife, Elizabeth, when he hitched a ride on a bus that she oversaw to transport patients. She told him if he sat in the back and kept quiet, he could come along. "And that was the story of the rest of my life," he said. They married during the blitz.

A bout of acute ulcerative colitis that nearly killed him derailed his plans to go into surgery after graduation, so he went into laboratory medicine instead, steered by an influential department chairman into microbiology. In the late 1940s, he worked with Dr. Mary Ethel Florey, a member of the team at Oxford who had developed penicillin for clinical use.

It was, he said, "a wildly exciting time" to be in infectious diseases. Penicillin was just coming into wider use and streptomycin was in testing.[31]

"We had a whole ward of paraplegic patients, mostly war casualties," he said. "These boys all got urinary tract infections, and in those days, they all pretty much died. We tried streptomycin when it came out to see whether that would be the magic medicine that would keep the infections at bay."

The magic medicine worked—briefly. But within weeks or days, the pathogens developed resistance. In the laboratory, the researchers could watch it happen in petri dishes.

"First, all of the organisms disappeared," Sherris said. "Then, very tiny, rather sickly colonies would develop in the individual patient [cultures]. You would see it on the plates. And then, a few days later, they were fully resistant. Some people at that time began to wonder whether we were going to have a window of use of antibiotics and then we were going to lose them all because of resistance."

Decades later, that fear would loom even larger.

But new antibiotics came through the pipeline, and the laboratory became involved early on in testing for susceptibility and resistance. Infections that had killed patients regularly, like streptococcal sepsis, were suddenly treatable.

Fast forward a decade, and Sherris was working in a laboratory in Manchester, England. His colleagues were excellent microbiologists, but he missed having a hand in clinical research. So he was intrigued when, in July 1958, Dr. Charles Evans, who had chaired the UW Department of Microbiology since the medical school's founding, stopped by between scientific meetings in London and Stockholm.

Evans had become involved in a national effort to upgrade clinical bacteriology, which had assumed new importance with the development of antibiotic therapy.[32] He sought out Sherris after reading his publications in laboratory management of infectious diseases as well as more fundamental research. Evans believed that recruiting Sherris to head the UW microbiology laboratory would position the university as a leader in laboratory development. He was right.

Sherris was already familiar with the UW because he had been following Kirby's research on antibiotic resistance in the medical literature, particularly his discovery of staphylococcal penicillinase. Soon Sherris was on his way to Seattle to "be inspected," as he put it. He met with just about everyone at the still-small school, which he found full of "fascinating personalities." It didn't hurt that the sun shone during his visit, and Mount Rainer was out. He spent a day with the Kirby family, who charmed him with their affability.

Many years later, after Kirby died, Sherris wrote to Kirby's three children that their father's "presence in Seattle was a major factor in my decision to come here, and it was he and your mother who welcomed us so warmly when we arrived and helped us get settled."[33]

By March 1959, John and Elizabeth Sherris had moved to Seattle, and he was installed as associate professor and head of the Clinical Microbiology Laboratories. He was back to working closely with clinicians, which he had missed in Manchester. He got along well with Kirby, whose dry humor Sherris appreciated, and often teamed up with him. Sherris soon landed the first NIH-funded university clinical laboratory postdoctoral training program grant.

Within a year, another fascinating personality would arrive. And the building would begin in earnest.

2

The

Early Years

Robert G. Petersdorf arrived in Seattle in 1960 with his wife, the former Patricia Horton Qua; the two had met and married at Yale, where she worked after graduating from the Yale School of Nursing. At 34, Petersdorf became the first chief of medicine at Harborview Medical Center.

Harborview became a clinical teaching site when the University of Washington School of Medicine enrolled its first class in 1946, but it had been around much longer than that. Originally opened in 1877 as King County Hospital, it was moved to its present location on Seattle's First Hill in 1931 and renamed for its view overlooking Puget Sound. Medical school faculty members commuted between their research laboratories on the university campus and their clinical activities and offices at Harborview until the university built a new hospital on the health sciences campus.[34]

Once the UW Medical Center opened in 1959, the initial faculty group took up full-time residence there. That's where Bill Kirby operated his lab and saw patients. John Sherris directed the clinical microbiology laboratories.

With the rest of the faculty decamped to the main campus, Petersdorf started with a clean slate. He also had the freedom to manage his own program, which suited his entrepreneurial style.[35] He set about establishing now-legendary standards for clinical care, teaching, and scholarship. In four years, he hired a dozen faculty members, essentially a department of medicine within the larger department.[36]

Under Petersdorf, Harborview became the site of a second group of infectious-diseases researchers. In time, it would grow to be larger than the group based at UW. Its champion was Marvin Turck, a physician-researcher who started out as Petersdorf's first fellow.

Turck first arrived in Seattle in 1960 more or less by accident, courtesy of the EIS, the disease-detective arm of the US Public Health Service. Founded in 1951, the highly selective postdoctoral training program based at the CDC in Atlanta put fellows through an epidemiology "boot camp" and then sent them out to work for two years in the field, investigating outbreaks and implementing control measures.

Petersdorf had asked if the EIS could send someone to set up a surveillance system at Harborview for infections caused by Gram-negative bacteria.[37] Turck, who was 26 at the time, later wrote that Petersdorf had been hoping for someone more seasoned than "some brash youngster from Chicago who had merely finished a year of internship."[38]

But Turck was no disappointment. Petersdorf, like his mentor, Paul Beeson, had an eye for talent. Soon enough, Turck began doing double duty as both an EIS officer and as Petersdorf's fellow.

A partnership began.

The overachiever: Marvin Turck

Chicago born and bred, Marvin Turck was a first-generation American and the first in his family of Eastern European immigrants to go on to college. He would joke that he had no choice but to go to medical school to fulfill his Jewish mother's dream, but in truth the vigorous premed courses at the Navy Pier Branch of the University of Illinois in Chicago appealed to his competitive spirit. "I have been overachieving since," he wrote.[39]

In his first week of medical school at the University of Illinois, he answered an ad for a student helper. He found himself working for the next four years in the Common Cold Laboratory of infectious-diseases researcher George G. Jackson.

"Thus began my own fledgling career in infectious diseases," Turck later wrote.[40] It was, he said, a "random and serendipitous" career launch. "Had I found a job in a different lab," he said, "I might have gone in a different direction."[41]

He found the people and the work agreeable, and, however serendipitous the choice, he forged ahead with characteristic intensity. In addition to working in Jackson's lab, Turck attended infectious-diseases rounds every Wednesday afternoon conducted by, among others, Harry F. Dowling, the chair of medicine. Dowling, renowned himself, had been the first of more than 100 "Finland Fellows" under legendary infectious-diseases physician-researcher Maxwell Finland of Harvard Medical School and Boston City Hospital.

By the time Turck had finished his medical degree, he felt that he had packed in the equivalent of a two-year infectious-diseases fellowship. Squeezing twice as much from every experience would become his custom.

Throughout both college and medical school, Turck pursued a second passion—and brought in extra income—by working as a stand-up comedian. It was a role he would reprise with relish throughout his long career, his Borscht Belt jokes as much a trademark as his deep clinical knowledge and skilled bedside teaching.

After graduating in 1959, Turck did a year of internship at the University of Illinois and published his first paper along with Dowling and other coauthors.[42] By then, he had reached the limits of his deferment from military service. To meet his obligation but avoid being sent to Korea, he applied to the EIS and was accepted into its 1960 class. Better to be a "shoe-leather epidemiologist," the term coined by EIS founder Alexander Langmuir, than a foot soldier, Turck wrote.[43]

He spent just six weeks in Atlanta. Having no more than finished the introductory EIS course, he received his first assignment: Seattle. Turck had married in medical school, and Seattle was a welcome destination for his wife, Rahla, whose sister and her family lived there. Over the years, Turck would recruit other promising EIS officers to continue their infectious-diseases research at the UW.

Little was known at that time about the epidemiology of Gram-negative organisms. In Jackson's lab during medical school, Turck had studied rhinovirus infections, with a bit of experience in Jackson's other research interest, UTIs. UTIs became his focus in Seattle.

Petersdorf, Turck wrote, gave him "laboratory space, a technician, a media maker, and full freedom to pursue my interests."[44] He took full advantage of those resources. In Turck's two years in Seattle, he published 12 papers on various aspects of Gram-negative infections.

After he completed his EIS service, Turck honored an obligation to return to Chicago in 1962 to be senior medical resident at the Research and Educational Hospital and the following year, chief medical resident at Cook County Hospital Service. There, under cardiologist Rolf Gunnar, he honed the clinical skills that would later establish his reputation as an inspiring teacher of bedside medicine.[45] He would soon take those skills back to Seattle.

The wizard: Seymour Klebanoff

While Petersdorf was building up his team of clinician-researchers at Harborview, the UW chair of medicine, Robert H. Williams, continued adding to the department overall. He had his eye on a promising researcher on an Arthritis and Rheumatism Fellowship at the Rockefeller Institute in New York and in 1962 recruited him to the UW. His name was Seymour J. Klebanoff.

Klebanoff was a wizard of a scientist. He was also a gentle colleague and a dedicated mentor, known as much for his kindness and incisive wit as for the considerable force of his scholarship. In time, he would take over from Kirby as head of the newly combined and renamed UW Division of Allergy and Infectious Diseases, leading it from 1976 to 1994.

Ask anyone about him, and the answer is the same: "We all loved Seymour." He was low-key and self-effacing—a great listener, not a huge talker. He was a careful, thoughtful, and efficient administrator, a "fatherly giant"[46] whose sense of fairness and equanimity many attributed to his Canadian upbringing.

Klebanoff was born in Toronto, Ontario, in 1927, to Samuel and Ann Klebanoff, who had emigrated to Canada from Belarus. He received his medical degree from the University of Toronto in 1951, coauthoring his first paper a year earlier. He earned a doctorate in biochemistry from University College London in 1954 and further trained as a fellow in pathological chemistry at the University of Toronto before going to the Rockefeller Institute.

His research focused on the immune system's chemical weapons against bacteria and viruses, particularly how white blood cells defend the body against bacterial infections. In 1967, he published a landmark study[47] describing how certain white blood cells called phagocytes produce an enzyme called myeloperoxidase that engulfs and destroys harmful bacteria.

"It's as if the phagocytes attract bacteria in an intracellular swimming pool and then turn on a spigot of Clorox to kill them," Klebanoff wrote.[48]

This discovery changed science's understanding of the body's natural defense mechanisms in fighting infections. Over the years, Klebanoff's research led to a better grasp of inflammation and host defense mechanisms and new insights and approaches for treating diseases in which immune responses are impaired. In 1978 he published "The Neutrophil: Function and Clinical Disorders" with his laboratory mentee, Robert Clark. The 600-page tome was widely considered the definitive reference.

He was a careful but efficient researcher, organizing his work into publications even before he began his experiments.

"Most of us kind of bumble along, get a whole bunch of data, and ask, 'How can we make this a publication?'" said Wes Van Voorhis, an infectious-diseases fellow under Klebanoff from 1986 to 1989 who went on to head the ID Division from 2007 to 2017. "Seymour would start thinking about a problem and write it out on lined sheets of yellow paper, then do the experiment and fill in the sheets. He would only do the experiments necessary to write the paper, while most of us would do way more than we needed to do."

Of course, the experiment wouldn't always go the way he wanted— that's the surprise of science. But with characteristic calm, Van Voorhis said, Klebanoff would redo the paper.

As a mentor, he was a wellspring of wisdom, dispensed in his typical low-key fashion. Van Voorhis recalled once fretting over whether to invest his time in applying for a grant that he may not get. Klebanoff said, "Look, Wes, if you don't apply for the grant, then you're surely not going to get it."

"It was sort of like Yogi Berra—so obvious it was funny," said Van Voorhis.

For all his self-effacement, Klebanoff's research earned him membership in the National Academy of Sciences and the Institute of

Medicine. Among his many awards were the MERIT Award from the NIH, the Alexander Fleming Award of the Infectious Disease Society of America, and the Bristol-Myers Squibb Award for distinguished achievement in infectious-diseases research. In 2007, he received the prestigious lifetime achievement award from the Association of American Medical Colleges for Distinguished Research in the Biomedical Sciences.

In addition to his research, mentoring and division leadership, his other UW responsibilities included serving as acting chair (1979-1980) and associate chair (1997-1999) of the Department of Medicine. He directed two major UW training programs: the Research Training Unit (1964-1976) and the Medical Scientist Training Program (1972-1977), in which a highly select group of students earn both MD and PhD degrees.

Petersdorf becomes chair of medicine

About the time Turck had headed back to Chicago, Petersdorf was promoted to full professor at age 36, after just two years at the UW. About two years after that, Robert H. Williams, who had become the UW's founding chair of medicine in 1948, suffered a heart attack and stepped down from his position. Petersdorf was named to succeed him in 1964, becoming, at age 38, one of the youngest chairs in the country.[49]

That Petersdorf rose so quickly was no surprise to Turck, who saw firsthand his skill and drive. Turck also believed that Petersdorf's specialization in infectious diseases played a role in his rise.

"Many of the people starting in infectious diseases became chiefs of medicine and other academic leadership positions," Turck said. "The mindset was different. A lot of that had to do with not having to be trained first in some kind of procedure. You had to do histories and physicals and be very thorough. You had to be interested in very cognitive things."[50]

(Turck's view that ID training was a gateway to academic leadership would prove true for generations of UW fellows, including one who would go on to become the senior executive leader of UW Medicine. Paul Ramsey arrived in Seattle as an ID fellow in 1978, during

Petersdorf's last years as chair. He became the department's third chair in 1990 and the first holder of the Robert G. Petersdorf Endowed Chair in Medicine, then rose to be vice president for medical affairs, dean of the UW School of Medicine, and CEO of the 26,000-employee healthcare system.)

Petersdorf would remain chair for 15 years, doing what he had done at Harborview on a much larger scale. In addition to his considerable administrative duties, in 1968 he began editing a major textbook, *Harrison's Principles of Internal Medicine*, which he would do for the next 22 years.

His growing national reputation as a clinician and his professional charisma attracted exceptional young physicians to Seattle—in those early days, mostly men—who would go on to become leaders in both infectious diseases and general internal medicine.

During his time as chair, Petersdorf grew the Department of Medicine from 69 full-time faculty members to 322, surpassing even the pace set under Beeson at Yale. (There had been 18 full-time faculty when Beeson arrived as chair in 1952 and 65 when he left, in 1965, to take a research post at Oxford.)[51] UW Medicine also added new divisions, which, with generous funding from the NIH, came to function as minidepartments.

Throughout most of Petersdorf's tenure, Bill Kirby headed the Division of Infectious Diseases.

"Because both he and I were infectious disease specialists, there could have been the opportunity for sibling rivalry," Petersdorf wrote years later in a tribute after Kirby died at age 82 in 1997. "It never happened. He was invariably kind and supportive. He never refused anything I asked him to do. Although we sometimes differed, we respected each other's work and clinical judgment."[52]

Kirby's daughter, Barbara Kirby, remembers how much her father admired Petersdorf's skill at managing arguments during committee and faculty meetings. During one such meeting, a knock-down, drag-out fight erupted between some members of the faculty and Petersdorf over the first item on the agenda. But when it was over, Petersdorf calmly said, "Let's go on to Item B," and continued as though nothing had happened.

"My dad had marveled at that," Barbara Kirby said. "He considered that an art. He said, 'I could not have done that—disagree mightily with someone and five minutes later, wipe the slate clean and approach a new topic.'

"I'm sure they had disagreements," she added. "I'm sure they argued about space and everything else, because as chairman, you make hard decisions. Bob Petersdorf was probably more forceful than Dad, but at heart, probably a pussycat."[53]

John Sherris, who knew and wrote papers with both, agreed that the two infectious-diseases experts got on well together. Harborview may have played a role in that. With Kirby running the full infectious-diseases division from the UW campus, Petersdorf, after becoming chair, kept a hand in ID research underway at Harborview. "I imagine Petersdorf used Harborview as a place where the young people he thought were promising and that he liked could go and get their training," Sherris said.[54]

In fact, he stationed one of his first hires there. Shortly after becoming chair of medicine, Petersdorf brought Turck back to Seattle as a UW assistant professor and chief of infectious diseases at Harborview. Turck was then 30 years old.

With Turck's installation, two arms of ID research arose. Kirby's arm, based on the UW health sciences campus, dealt primarily with antibiotics. The Harborview arm over time would grow both larger and more diverse.

The Kirby-Bauer test

Although Turck worked primarily with Petersdorf, he also worked with Kirby to build on a project already underway. It would lead to one of medicine's most widely cited papers and widely used tests, the Kirby-Bauer test.

Kirby had done some of the earliest studies of resistance to antibiotics. If the wonder drugs were to remain effective, their use needed to be managed carefully. It became obvious to Kirby that a simple test was needed to determine a pathogen's susceptibility or resistance before prescribing an antibiotic.

He began working to develop one in the late 1950s, joined in the effort by his 1959–1960 research fellow Alfred Bauer. Bauer graduated from medical school in Germany in 1953 and moved to the United

States in 1956, doing postgraduate studies until he qualified to practice medicine here. (He did not stay in infectious diseases, going on to become a pediatrician in Seattle and in Kirkland, Washington.)[55]

The standardized, single-disk-diffusion method they developed—still used worldwide today— uses small disks of filter paper impregnated with different antibiotics. These are placed onto agar plates where bacteria are growing. If an antibiotic prevents the growth of the bacteria strain, a clear ring or "zone of inhibition" can be observed around it. Bacteria can be identified as susceptible, intermediate, or resistant to antibiotics being tested depending on the size of the zone, if there is one.

It was simple—and brilliant. Before, testing involved growing bacteria in five or six test tubes with different concentrations of a single antibiotic to see which if any dose was effective. It was time-consuming and expensive. The Kirby-Bauer test was simple enough to be done even in small hospitals and clinics around the world.

Kirby worked for years to refine the technique—testing various antibiotics against various bacteria using exactly the same method, time after time, measuring zone widths and cut-off points for susceptibility. Sherris, who had been involved in susceptibility-and-resistance testing from early in his career, joined him and was especially diligent at documenting the advantages of the single-disk method to other tests. When Turck came to the UW, he got involved by testing the method on Gram-negative pathogens as well as the Gram-positive bacteria Kirby and Bauer had used.

In 1966, the paper describing the test was published in the *American Journal of Clinical Pathology* with Bauer, Kirby, Sherris, and Turck as authors. After many hearings, the Food and Drug Administration in 1972 published the method in the Federal Register, and in 1975 it became the basis of the National Committee for Clinical Laboratory Standards disk diffusion standards. Sherris worked with Swedish researchers to coordinate efforts of an international group to recommend the method as well.

"Our paper has been widely cited because it was the definitive and detailed description, incorporating earlier contributions by us and others, of a simple, efficient, and practical way of measuring clinically applicable susceptibility of bacteria to a number of antimicrobial agents simultaneously," Kirby wrote.[56]

In his personal life, however, Kirby remained typically low-key about "that thing he was famous for," as his children, who all went on to become physicians, recalled. Years later, when his daughter, Barbara, was in medical school, she learned about the Kirby-Bauer test for the first time when she took a microbiology class under Sherris.

"He really was modest," Barbara Kirby said of her father. "He would have been a billionaire if he had patented the test, even if he got a zillionth of a penny for every test done. But he said no, he didn't care about that. He was all about the science, about contributing what he could."[57]

Turck's first fellow: Allan Ronald

Turck continued with his primary research into UTIs. He particularly drilled down into *Escherichia coli*, a rod-shaped, Gram-negative bacterium first discovered by Theodor Escherich in 1885 and a common cause of UTIs. Petersdorf maintained an interest in the subject and shared authorship on the early papers coming out of Turck's lab, but "did not hinder me or my identity," Turck said.[58] As a mentor, Petersdorf steered Turck toward involvement in the right academic organizations, such as the fledgling Infectious Diseases Society of America, of which Petersdorf, Beeson, and Kirby were charter members. And, of course, the Pus Club.

What Turck loved most—and what he and others agreed he did best—was teach.

"Many of us have strengths in different areas," Turck said. "My major forte was teaching infectious diseases."[59]

Like Petersdorf, Turck had an eye for talent.

"I started with very good people," he said. "The secret to being a good mentor is to start with good mentees. You have to be able to select good people and hope that they will eventually exceed the teacher. That happened in Seattle."[60]

Turck took enormous satisfaction in the accomplishments of his fellows and chief residents as they developed into academic and clinical leaders. Dozens went on to attain international recognition. Just as he felt proud of being Petersdorf's first fellow, he took particular pride in his own first fellow, Allan Ronald, and first chief resident, King Holmes.

Ronald met Petersdorf and Turck in 1964. Petersdorf was still in his early days as chair of medicine, and Turck had just returned to Seattle to head infectious diseases at Harborview.

A young Canadian medical school graduate who had won a medal for top marks in what at the time was called bacteriology at the University of Manitoba, Ronald wanted to pursue training in infectious diseases. He looked south because, he said, "I realized Americans were teaching a lot of things we weren't in Canada."[61]

His first stop had been a two-year fellowship at the University of Maryland under Dr. Theodore E. Woodward, who founded and led one of the first ID divisions in the world, established in 1948 (a year ahead of Bill Kirby, albeit in a medical school that was 140 years older than the UW).[62] Like Beeson, Kirby, and Petersdorf, Woodward was a charter member of the Infectious Diseases Society of America.

Ronald recalls him as a strong teacher and role model with a soft Southern drawl. Hospitals were still segregated when Ronald arrived in June 1962 and was assigned to oversee a ward of African-American women. He practically lived at the hospital, so intent was he on giving them the best care. After a month, he called his girlfriend, Myrna, a nurse, and said, "I need you here." His short trip back to Winnipeg for the wedding launched a lifelong partnership.

Woodward, who published papers with Petersdorf and coedited the infectious-diseases portion of the classic *Harrison's* medical text, recommended Seattle as Ronald's next stop. "He told me he was going to pass me on to Dr. Petersdorf because he very highly respected the Seattle program," Ronald recalled.

But just as he and Myrna were preparing to move, Woodward asked if he would first help open a research program in Lahore, Pakistan. The 10 months he and Myrna spent there—and the lessons learned in what to do or not to do in a different culture—would stand him in good stead for the groundbreaking work he later launched in sub-Saharan Africa.

"It's about understanding the culture and being humble and working alongside these very bright individuals," he said. "In that way, we were successful." The program on maternal and child health that he helped establish in Lahore continues today.

That first Seattle meeting was just to get acquainted before Pakistan. Ronald returned to the UW in July 1965 to become Turck's first fellow.

"We rarely saw Petersdorf because he was so engaged in the politics of medicine and in being who he was, an exemplary leader," said Ronald. "Marvin was incredibly busy too, but he was very committed to my establishing myself, and thanks to him, I did establish myself as an investigator. He was very, very bright and a good role model. It was a privilege to be Marvin's fellow."

Turck was still early in his own career. The two of them, he told Ronald, would be writing lots of manuscripts.

"We worked hard," Ronald said. "We learned a lot that wasn't known about urinary tract infections. And we wrote manuscripts and got them published in good journals. Marvin told me, 'You're going to learn about infections all your life, but you're only going to learn research over the next couple of years. That is the priority: to learn how to do research, to learn how to establish yourself in your area.'"

Turck also showed him how to organize clinical trials, introduced him to CDC researchers in Atlanta, and taught him advanced clinical skills. He was both a great clinician and a great teacher, Ronald said. "He had a story to tell of every patient he saw, and the stories lived on in your way of thinking, he told them so well. He had 1,000 stories."

During his second year at the UW, Ronald worked for two months in Sherris's microbiology laboratory. "I loved the way that John Sherris did things," he said. "That's when I decided I should do that as well as infectious diseases."

It would be microbiology that took him back to Canada. None of the academic medical centers Ronald contacted in Canada were interested in hiring an infectious-diseases specialist. Sentiment was growing that the era of infectious diseases was over. Public sanitation, vaccines, and antibiotics had won the day. So Ronald returned to Seattle and spent a full year in Sherris's laboratory, training in clinical microbiology.

"I went to Winnipeg in 1968 as a microbiologist," he said. "That's what they wanted."

But Ronald was neither convinced the war against infectious diseases was over nor deterred in his ambition to replicate Seattle's infectious-diseases program at his new home at the University of Manitoba.[63] He continued his research into the management of UTIs, started an infection control program, and improved antimicrobial use and oversight. Over the next decade, he worked with public health officials to investigate outbreaks of infectious diseases, often consulting with Turck or his contacts at the CDC. He and Turck continued to write papers together about the outbreak investigations, two of which were published in the *New England Journal of Medicine*. Over the next 50 years, Ronald would train almost 100 physicians from across Canada and the world in infectious diseases, drawing on the training he had received in Seattle.

In 1975, Winnipeg experienced a huge chancroid outbreak. That investigation and its aftermath would lead Ronald to a global career and a key partnership with another mentee of Turck's that Turck took particular pride in—his first chief resident, King Holmes.

3

Becoming a Force

Born in Saint Paul, Minnesota, in 1937, King Kennard Holmes was named for his paternal grandfather, Wesley E. King, whose architectural and engineering firm—Tolz, King & Day—designed roads, bridges, mass transit, and iconic buildings: the Cathedral of Saint Paul, the Union Depot headquarters of the Great Northern and the Northern Pacific railroads, and the Prince of Wales Hotel in Canada's Waterton Lakes National Park.

As a freshman at Harvard, Holmes thought he, too, would be an architect until he met a fellow student with similar ambitions—and a much better hand at drawing. He decided on medicine even before realizing that it, too, would allow him to build.

He earned his medical degree from Cornell University Medical College in 1963 and did his internship at Vanderbilt University Medical Center in Nashville, Tennessee. At Vanderbilt, he was assigned, purely by chance, to the microbiology laboratory for his first rotation.

With no knowledge of infectious diseases or inkling that it would become his career, he threw himself into identifying microbes and testing for resistance. He all but moved in, working every day and often into the night—a pattern that would stay with him for a lifetime. And because he and his wife could eat for free at the hospital, they took breakfast, lunch, and dinner there, stretching a monthly paycheck that just barely covered the rent on their Nashville house.

Others in the lab, who were farther along in their training, warned Holmes against getting too invested.

"They said, 'Don't go into this field. We've got antibiotics for everything now. We're not going to have an infectious disease field anymore,'" Holmes recalled. "I was a little discouraged."[64]

But he was proud when Dr. David E. Rogers, Vanderbilt's head of medicine, gave grand rounds using data from the work he had done in the lab. From that came his first published paper, analyzing the antimicrobial patterns for all of the isolates that came into the laboratory.

He presented the sixty-page draft to Rogers over dinner at the faculty club. Rogers, who would go on to be the first head of the Robert Wood Johnson Foundation and a national leader in fighting AIDS, deftly shortened it to three pages before its publication in the Southern Medical Journal.

Holmes's next move would have an even greater influence on his career. It was 1964, and although combat troops were not yet on the ground, the US presence in South Vietnam was growing. The US Navy drafted Holmes under the so-called "doctor draft," which had been in place since the 1950s to channel physicians into two-year service in the Army, the Navy, the Air Force, or the Public Health Service. He was to be stationed at the Naval Air Weapons Station in California's Mojave Desert.

To a Minnesota native, that sounded awfully hot.

Holmes asked his detail officer for an assignment at a research laboratory or teaching hospital, preferably one in Hawaii or Japan. In exchange, he offered to stay on with the Navy for a third year. The Navy captain barked back, "Well, okay. If we do this, I'd be watching you. If you didn't sign up for a third year, I'm shipping your ass to Vietnam, boy."[65] Holmes reassured him that he would, his trademark calm and low-key banter already in evidence. Before the conversation ended, he was being called "son" instead of "boy." He shipped out to Honolulu.

Within a year, he became the epidemiologist for the US 7th Fleet, the Navy's largest, with an area of operations spanning the Western Pacific and Indian oceans. Getting—and then doing—the job involved both luck and pluck.

Assigned at first to the dispensary at Pearl Harbor, Holmes found himself working extra shifts to fill in for a physician named David

Johnson. After six months, he finally bumped into Johnson at the officers' club bar and, wondering why Johnson was never around, asked what he did. Johnson replied that he went out on the ships, investigating disease outbreaks. He was the fleet's epidemiologist.

Intrigued, Holmes said, "If it ever opens up, I would love to have that job."

Shortly afterward, Johnson called Holmes. "Were you serious?" he asked. Johnson had just been promoted to director of the Preventive Medicine Unit—and offered to make Holmes the head of epidemiology.

Not that Holmes had ever studied epidemiology.

After enthusiastically accepting, Holmes hustled over to the University of Hawaii to learn about his new field. The first person he encountered was Clair E. Folsome, his former lab instructor from his Harvard undergraduate days, whose class he had, in his own words, bombed. But Folsome, a visionary whose experiments with sealed, palm-sized globes of tiny shrimp, algae, and microbes would later inspire Biosphere II,[66] saw promise in Holmes and agreed to be his microbiology mentor.

Fulsome introduced Holmes to Dr. Robert Worth, a leprosy expert, whose fieldwork took him to Micronesia, New Guinea, Hong Kong, and Nepal and whose research helped end the confinement of Hansen's disease patients on the island of Molokai. Modest and unimposing despite his international reputation, Worth became Holmes's mentor in epidemiology.

Every day, Holmes would go into his office at the preventive medicine clinic to check reports coming in from the fleet. Then he surfed in the late afternoons off Waikiki Beach, had dinner with his wife and their then only child, and headed for classes in the evening.

His PhD thesis committee included O.A. Bushnell, a microbiologist, medical historian, and best-selling novelist whose last book, *The Gifts of Civilization: Germs and Genocide in Hawaii*, is considered the definitive study of how Native Hawaiians were nearly wiped out by newly introduced tuberculosis, smallpox, leprosy, and STDs. Bushnell's literary chops were as much a draw as his microbiology skills to Holmes, who considered his first mentor to be the high school English teacher who had assigned him to read a book a day.

When it came to choosing a thesis topic, another mentor—virologist and dengue expert Leon Rosen—offered this advice: Choose a topic that's not going to go away, that you can work on for the rest of your life.

Holmes's topic more or less chose him, but the choice fit Rosen's standard. On his first day as fleet epidemiologist, Holmes arrived at his desk to find 30 reports of incurable gonorrhea.[67] STDs, he figured, were not likely to go away.

US military records on STDs date back to the Revolutionary War. In World War I—before the availability of antibiotics—only the great influenza pandemic of 1918–1919 accounted for more loss of service days than STDs.[68]

So, not surprisingly, military researchers have made significant contributions over the years to the understanding of, prevention, and treatment of these diseases. During World War II, US Army investigators published the first large-scale trial of penicillin treatment for gonorrhea. An unpublished clinical trial conducted during the Korean War found that infections were reduced by giving penicillin to troops prophylactically before leave periods.[69]

And during the Vietnam era, a young Navy lieutenant who talked his way into becoming the epidemiologist of the 7th Fleet while simultaneously getting his PhD in epidemiology set standards for the epidemiology and management of gonococcal infections that are still in use today.

Going out on the USS Enterprise, Holmes set up a research project in Olongapo City, Philippines, northwest of Manila and next to Subic Bay, a deep-water port at which Navy vessels docked. Along with about 200 bars, Olongapo had more than 5,000 "registered hostesses," prostitution being technically illegal. An average of 50 percent of the sailors taking shore leave there developed "the drip." When King first became fleet epidemiologist and saw those reports of treatment-resistant gonorrhea, standard treatment was to treat any urethral discharge with a recommended dose of penicillin. Only about half the men responded.

No one was analyzing the discharge, so Holmes took swabs and froze them to take back to the laboratory he had by then set up back in Hawaii. About half turned out to be gonorrhea, and testing showed increased resistance to the penicillin dose they were given. The rest Holmes identified as nongonococcal urethritis syndrome, which was not sensitive to penicillin.

He designed a clinical trial that found that adding probenecid to the standard penicillin dose raised the cure rate. Later, he tried tetracycline, which took care of both the gonorrhea and the non-gonococcal infections.

"What we found was that there was resistance, and the resistant strains were responsive to this new approach to treatment," he said. "But we also found that it wasn't all gonorrhea. Half of it was another infection that they weren't detecting. And it was happening all throughout the Pacific."[70]

Holmes didn't stop with the sailors. On his next trip, he met with the Olongapo Bar Owners Association—a meeting memorialized in a seedy-looking photo—to ask about medical care for the sex workers. The city supported a clinic, overseen by a Filipino *doctora* whom the ever-affable Holmes befriended. She invited Holmes to observe while she treated 250 women a day, using—as Holmes witnessed—a single plastic speculum.

"I thought to myself, 'Hmmm, that might be one reason there's a lot of gonorrhea occurring,'" he said.[71] And while the *doctora* used the right stain to test for gonorrhea, the treatment she used—a formulation of penicillin called benzathine that persists in low concentrations in the body—was practically designed to create resistance.

Holmes brought in hundreds of metal speculums and an autoclave to sterilize them. Working with the *doctora*, he began testing 500 women a day and treating those who had gonorrhea with ampicillin. On the first day, a couple of women fainted, and he feared they had had allergic reactions to the drug. But it turned out that the women, waiting their turn in the auditorium where he'd set up shop, had just panicked. Someone got the idea to bring in giant dolls to comfort nerves. It worked, making the women laugh. Holmes and the *doctora* tested and treated thousands of women.

The incidence of gonorrhea following shore leave in Olongapo fell to about 5 percent. "King Holmes should have received the Congressional Medal of Honor!" wrote Dr. David A. Schwartz, Holmes's successor as fleet epidemiologist.[72]

The lesson Holmes took from the experience was this: "The key thing is to get out into the field and find out what's happening—why they are finding antibiotic resistance, or whatever the problem," he said. "You can't sit back in the laboratory and test strains and figure out why people are resistant. You have to see why."[73]

Looking back from the vantage of 50 years to his career's unlikely launch, he added, "When you suddenly acquire more responsibility than you might in a real-life situation, it's transforming."[74]

He would later seek to bestow that kind of transforming experience on his own mentees, who numbered more than 150, sending them out into the world to build a network, a way of doing things, and a body of knowledge as lasting and influential as any his grandfather designed.

Holmes finished his three-year commitment in 1967 with a PhD and a string of publications. During those years, he also made a contact that would help determine where he went next. Concern that treating the women might trigger an adverse reaction, he had sought advice from a source who was relatively nearby—Paul P. Van Arsdel, Jr., who had joined the faculty of the University of Washington in 1954 as its first head of the Division of Allergy.

The UW, King heard, also was developing a reputation for infectious-diseases research.

The move to Seattle

Three years of active duty behind him, Holmes moved to Seattle to start his residency at the University of Washington. Petersdorf had been chair of medicine for three years. Turck was still chief of infectious diseases at Harborview but would soon take on a new position as chief of medicine at another UW clinical teaching site, the US Public Health Service Hospital.

Holmes's first meeting with Petersdorf came when the chair invited the house staff—including newly arriving interns, residents, and fellows—to his home for a summer party. Holmes had been tending to a patient and arrived late. As he walked in the front door, he spotted a waiter hired for the party carrying what appeared to be the last bottle of wine back into the kitchen.

He followed.

Noting where the waiter put the bottle, Holmes pulled over a chair from the kitchen table and stepped up on it to reach the cabinet. He was just pulling the bottle out when Petersdorf walked into the kitchen.

"I said, 'I had a late patient, but I didn't want to miss your famous wine,'" Holmes said. "I poured myself a glass, stepped down from the chair, and went in and talked to everybody."[75]

He made a lasting impression. Petersdorf asked Holmes to do teaching rounds on papers he had published during his Navy years. He also invited the young physician-researcher to Atlantic City to attend the annual meeting of the American Society for Clinical Investigation, which held a dinner for its infectious-diseases subgroup. Petersdorf was a prominent figure in those meetings and his protege, Marvin Turck, was becoming prominent as well.

During his first year of residency, Holmes found an informal mentor in Sherrill J. Slichter, who was doing a UW fellowship in hematology and oncology. In her long career, Slichter went on to make significant contributions to transfusion medicine, leading long-term studies that extended storage time of platelets and prevented transfused platelets from being rejected. She would later head the Bloodworks Northwest Research Institute.

"She taught me how to do everything," Holmes said. "I was doing bone marrow biopsies and stuff you don't usually get to do when you're a resident. She treated us like we were faculty members, not just residents. She was one of my heroes."[76]

A year in, Holmes decided he wanted to pursue further training in infectious diseases. And he had seen enough of Turck to know that he wanted Turck as his mentor.

"Marv was obviously smart and enthusiastic, and he really knew infectious diseases in a way I hadn't even been thinking about before," Holmes said. "So, I just said, 'Could I do a fellowship with you?'"[77]

But Turck told Holmes no, he wasn't taking on fellows because he was starting a new position as chief of medicine at the Public Health Service Hospital.

Holmes was undeterred by Turck's rejection and determined to follow him to the imposing art deco building looming over Seattle's downtown and visible from Harborview.

Originally part of the US Marine Hospital Service, the Public Health Service Hospital moved from Port Townsend to the then-newly constructed 312-bed facility on Beacon Hill in 1933. Marine hospitals had been established in 1798 to serve sick and disabled seaman and to perform health inspections of newly arriving immigrants. Over the years, the mandate was expanded to include care for Native

Americans, Alaska Natives, the poor and indigent, and, after World War I, injured veterans.

In 1951, marine hospitals were redesignated US Public Health Service hospitals. That same year, a VA hospital opened in Seattle. Robert Williams, the medical school's founding chair of medicine, arranged for each to be clinical teaching sites, along with Harborview. By the time Turck became its chief of medicine, the Public Health Service Hospital had by far the largest university teaching involvement of any PHS hospital in the nation.[78]

Holmes met with Petersdorf and with the director of UW's residency program about his plans. Before long, he became not Turck's fellow but his first chief resident.

"He was gracious about it," he said of Turck. "He said, 'OK, your office is going to be right next to mine.' So, I went over to the medical center to see the office right next to his, and it was a giant men's restroom."[79]

Holmes moved in.

Turck would become as proud of his first chief resident as he had been of his first fellow, Allan Ronald, who had completed his two-year fellowship and was at that time training with John Sherris. But it took some time for Turck and Holmes to bond.

During the morning report, in which the house staff updated the chief of medicine on newly admitted patients and other developments, Turck—whose sharp mind was always ahead of everyone's—had a habit of guessing what the residents were going to say and finishing their sentences. Holmes and other residents decided that, for all his jokes, the new chief of medicine needed to lighten up.

One morning, one of Holmes's coconspirators began filling Turck in on an urgent new case: A man who had been brought into the medical center by helicopter during the night from a Russian submarine. (That should have been enough to give the joke away, but no.) The patient was in and out of consciousness and running a high fever, the resident said, then went on to describe symptoms of pyelonephritis, a severe kidney infection, along with treatment with a drug they all knew Turck would find totally inappropriate.

Sure enough, before the resident had finished his report, Turck ran out the door, saying "Where is he? We've got to see him right now." Everyone fell into line after him and entered the patient's hospital room just as a nurse—who was in on the gag—was pulling a sheet over the man in the bed. Turck went up to the bed and began to shake the body under the sheet, saying "Son, son, are you OK?"

The body rose slowly—it was another of the residents.

"Keep in mind we were trying to teach him to not jump all over these cases and just let us finish up what the report is," Holmes said. "Marv looks at me and goes like this." Holmes banged his hand on his desk. "He knew what we were doing. And he took it a lot cooler after that."[80]

The joke was actually straight out of Turck's lesson book. Holmes credited Turck with teaching him that laughter helped defuse stressful situations. Although Holmes didn't try to repeat the stand-up routine that Turck was known for, he sought to do the same thing in his own deadpan way.

"What I learned from Marvin was the importance of humor," he said. "The bigger the challenge, the funnier the humor needs to be."[81]

Early on, Holmes came to know another UW researcher who had research space and offices at the Public Health Service Hospital. Dr. E. Donnall Thomas had arrived in Seattle from the Mary Imogene Bassett Hospital in Cooperstown, New York, in late 1963 to pursue research into the fledgling field of bone marrow transplantation to cure blood and immune system cancers. Most other investigators had abandoned the field after the first wave of experimental transplants in humans ended in the deaths of all patients from complications. But Thomas persisted, turning his studies to dogs when he first arrived in Seattle. A Cobalt-60 machine used to irradiate dogs before transplant was housed in an old bunker in West Seattle. [82]

In 1969, after performing transplants on 1,500 dogs with lymphoma, Thomas and his team received NIH funding to begin human transplants. The procedure used radiation and chemotherapy to destroy patients' diseased bone marrow, leaving them with no immune system until their new one took root. Many of the early deaths were due to infections by pathogens that would have been harmless in a healthy person.

Thomas was famously particular about whom he trusted to see his patients. Holmes was the first and for a while only infectious-diseases specialist called in to consult on the pathogens that preyed on the immune-suppressed.

"I consulted on all the people who developed complications," said Holmes. "That was a tough time for everybody."[83]

In those early days, the still experimental treatment was only attempted in patients with advanced leukemia, and most died from recurrent cancer or from complications of the transplant, including infections. But the team pressed on. And in time, infectious-diseases specialists would come to play a key role.

George Counts and Harry Beaty

Holmes was not the only physician-researcher drawn to the UW to study under Marvin Turck. At the time Holmes was starting his chief residency, another young physician-researcher who would play a role in UW's infectious-diseases division was just beginning his ID fellowship. George W. Counts came to Seattle because of Turck.

Born in 1935 in Idabel, Oklahoma, Counts was the son of sharecroppers who grew cotton and other crops. When he was 10, the family moved to Oklahoma City, settling in a close-knit community where everyone watched over each other's children. At age 18, Counts had been one of four black students to enroll in the University of Oklahoma. [84]

The push to integrate predated the Supreme Court's 1954 Brown v. Board of Education decision and was led by local black leaders, teachers, and parents, including his own, who wanted a better life for their son.

Counts studied chemical engineering, not so much by choice but because he was only allowed to attend the University of Oklahoma if he majored in a subject not taught at the local black college. He struggled the first year, with no help from the aloof counselor assigned to him. Wanting to make his family proud—and not be relegated to a life as a laborer—he came back the next year resolved to find a major that suited him better.

A course in plant sciences introduced him to bacteriology, as microbiology was then known. That became his passion and his major, influenced in no small part by the nurturing he received from Howard Larsh, the chairman of the Department of Plant Science. Larsh's interest and support helped to restore Counts's faith in his academic abilities after that discouraging first year, and he graduated with a BS in 1957. (In 2006, the University of Oklahoma gave him its Distinguished Alumnus award.)

He stayed on for a master's degree after receiving a graduate teaching assistantship. He found teaching, advising, and mentoring to be especially satisfying. "Decades later, I can still recall what a pleasure it was to help students master a simple skill such as viewing bacteria on a microscope slide and see the wonders that it first held for them," he wrote.[85]

Counts had planned to go for a doctorate, but Larsh urged him to get a medical degree instead. At medical school at the University of Iowa, Counts realized that he loved treating patients as much as he loved teaching. Graduating in 1965, he completed his internship and residency in internal medicine at the Ohio State University in Columbus. Then, with his keen interest in microbiology, he decided to apply for a postdoctoral fellowship in infectious diseases.

He wrote to seven or eight schools, including the UW. Turck responded with particular enthusiasm.

One year and one day older than Counts, Turck welcomed him as both a colleague and friend. He dazzled Counts with his clinical knowledge and skills and invited him to his son's bar mitzvah.

"He was extraordinary in so many ways," Counts said of Turck. "He had such a commitment to science and infectious diseases, and to sharing his knowledge. He was a generous man. And he was really sharp. He could name cases in an obscure journal no one else remembered. Throughout this he also had a commitment to serving as an attending physician."[86]

But because Turck was just taking on his new job as chief of medicine, he assigned Counts to the man who had succeeded him as chief of infectious diseases at Harborview: Harry Beaty, a leading researcher in bacterial meningitis.

Born in Brookfield, Missouri, in 1932, Harry Nelson Beaty worked his way through undergraduate and medical school at the UW, finishing his MD in 1958. After interning at the University of Minnesota, he spent three years in the Navy, then returned to the UW for his residency in internal medicine and training in infectious diseases.

He left again to do a post-doctoral fellowship in medicine and biochemistry at the NIH from 1963 to 1965, returning again, at

Petersdorf's invitation this time, to join the faculty. In 1968, Beaty took over from Turck as head of infectious diseases at Harborview, a position he would hold until 1975.

Beaty served with Petersdorf and Kirby on an advisory committee to Fort Lewis—the nearby US Army Base—on meningococcal disease. When five recruits developed sulfa-resistant meningitis and one of them died, Counts worked with Beaty to investigate whether minocycline given prophylactically could prevent a larger outbreak. Other drugs being tested elsewhere had failed, but minocycline bought Ft. Lewis enough time to vaccinate incoming recruits and for protection to be conferred from the polysaccharide vaccine then available, arresting the outbreak.[87]

Beaty was known as an excellent clinician with a breadth and depth of knowledge about medicine in general, not just infectious diseases.

"He was quiet," said Counts. "He had a good sense of humor, though he was not flashy or exuberant like Marvin."[88] But then, who could match Turck's stand-up routine?

Counts loved working at Harborview, and by the time he finished his fellowship, he'd fallen in love with Seattle.

But his career, at least temporarily, took him elsewhere. He took a position as an assistant professor at the University of Miami in the pathology and medicine departments and soon was asked to run the microbiology lab at Jackson Memorial Hospital. But that was not the last he saw of Turck and Seattle. When Beaty left Harborview to be chair of medicine at the University of Vermont (he would finish out his career as dean of the medical school at Northwestern University in Chicago), Turck lured Counts back to Seattle to take over as ID chief.

King's first fellow, Paul Wiesner

Another young physician-researcher drawn to Seattle because of Turck was Paul Wiesner. Turck assigned him to be Holmes's first fellow.

Holmes had finished up his year as Turck's chief resident and became head of infectious diseases and assistant chief of medicine at the Public Health Service Hospital. He continued the work he had begun in the Navy on STDs. Soon it became apparent that this field, once relegated to military researchers, was in high demand.

"There had been the introduction of oral contraceptives, the war going on in Southeast Asia, the baby boom coming of age, so there were many young adults who were sexually active," he said. "And so all of that came together in the '60s, and there were huge increases in STD epidemics."[89]

And he was practically the only person in the country working on it.

"It just seemed like a mission to help create a field that would take on this problem," he said. "The real challenge was finding resources, first, and then attracting new people into the field and overcoming the stigma of dealing with it."[90]

His first fellow appeared to be an unlikely candidate.

Paul Joseph Wiesner was born in 1940 in Neenah, Wisconsin, the fourth of seven sons of an athletic, civic-minded, and very Catholic family. He studied to be a priest, entering the Catholic Maryknoll Seminary after his sophomore year in high school, but eventually left for the University of Wisconsin. There he majored in philosophy before going on to earn a medical degree. He did his internship and residency in internal medicine at the University of Rochester.

For their first meeting in 1970, Wiesner went to Holmes's office. The younger man looked confused. It was a nice, big office—for an old men's room.

Holmes watched Wiesner take it all in—the tile walls, the little stalls.

"I could see him start to turn pale," Holmes said. "He said, 'What do you work on?' And I said, 'I work on gonorrhea research.' And he had just come out of a seminary and just about fainted."

Wiesner was about to get a very different education.

4

Shaping a

New Field

Although syphilis and gonorrhea had long been a concern, especially within the military, STD rates nationwide declined dramatically after penicillin came into use in the years following World War II. Many health authorities assumed the problem was solved.

That complacency lasted only 15 years. But during those post-war decades, once-vibrant academic programs in syphilis and other STDs shifted their emphasis elsewhere. Public STD clinics were neglected and underfunded. In many clinics nationwide, the supervising physicians were retired from previous careers and often only superficially engaged with and at times even hostile to STDs and the patients who had them. At the state and county level, STD-control programs had been largely dismantled or restricted to prostitutes.[91]

So it was little wonder that Paul Wiesner was taken aback to find that he would be studying STDs under King Holmes. As Holmes's second fellow, H. Hunter Handsfield, put it, "STDs were a backwater, intellectually and socially. No one cared about the people who got those problems, and there were no institutions with the interest and capability to study these things."[92]

Holmes was changing that. The drug resistance that he had seen firsthand during his Navy days told him that the gonorrhea problem was not solved. And the problem wasn't confined to the military or to sex workers and other stigmatized populations. In the late 1960s, after a decade of decline, gonorrhea and syphilis rates began to soar again, driven by the pill, the sexual awakening of the baby boom generation, and related social changes. In addition, Holmes had begun to track the high frequency of other conditions not yet widely understood to be sexually transmitted, such as nongonococcal urethritis, genital herpes, genital warts, and more.

"All of a sudden people say, 'Oops, we've got a problem,'" said Handsfield. "And a very small number of institutions said, 'OK, this is a niche we can fill.' The University of Washington was one of them. You've got a King Holmes—with the support of a Marvin Turck, a Bob Petersdorf, and a Bill Kirby—to say, 'Let's start developing the science, the modern microbiology, the virology in STDS.'"

And so began the modern era of STD research, with the UW on the ground floor. Throughout medical history, STD research had largely been limited to observational studies of clinical manifestations and treatment, with little emphasis on microbiology, virology, and immunology. That was about to change.

The clinical epidemiologist: Hunter Handsfield

H. Hunter Handsfield's interest in medicine began at age 11 when a drunk driver in his hometown of Garden City, Long Island, careened off the road and plowed into a group of kids playing in the parking strip. He was one of those kids. No one was killed, but he spent six weeks hospitalized and in traction and another three months in a body cast, which had to be patched several times—until his orthopedist spotted him batting baseballs and causing the damage to the cast.

Some people would never want to see a doctor again after such an experience. But the immersion in medicine fascinated the young Handsfield. That and his love of biology sealed his decision to go to medical school at Columbia University in New York City. His choice was strongly supported by his highly intellectual family, including his mother; her mother, one of the first female members of Phi Beta Kappa and a published feminist philosopher of the early twentieth century; and his father, then editor in chief of McGraw Hill's College Textbook Division, who had recruited economist Paul Samuelson and chemist Linus Pauling to write their famous textbooks.

Handsfield started his UW internship when Robert Petersdorf had been chair of medicine for four years and already was recognized nationwide as a leader in the field. Young physicians in training learned by taking care of patients but also by presenting cases in a formal setting and receiving a public critique. The level of anxiety involved depended on who was giving the critique. Some professors could be biting. Others were softer.

Petersdorf was both.

Once, Handsfield said, a medical student—let's call him Jones—stumbled in his presentation and was unable to answer first one then another of Petersdorf's questions. "Jones, I thought that if I led you to the edge of the cliff you might slip and fall over," Petersdorf said. A pause, and then: "But not you, Jones. You *dove*."

It was said with a broad grin and a twinkle in his eye, then the chair went on to list the good parts of Jones's presentation.

"He had this gruff exterior, and he'd make criticisms tinged with humor," Handsfield said. "Then he'd make very supportive comments. He was a great teacher."[93]

It was during Handsfield's residency that Petersdorf became one of the editors of *Harrison's Principles of Internal Medicine*. One morning during the residents' daily report to the chief, Petersdorf complained that the newly published edition had not yet arrived at the UW medical bookstore. Handsfield mentioned his father's senior position with McGraw Hill, the publisher. "See what you can do, Handsfield," came the wry reply.

Several days later, a shipment of ten books arrived. But it was even better than that. Petersdorf had long had a friendly rivalry with another editor, Maxwell Wintrobe, his counterpart as chair of medicine at the University of Utah; it turned out that the University of Utah's shipment had been diverted to Seattle, and Wintrobe was without his books for another week.

For the rest of his residency, ID fellowship, and for many years afterward, Handsfield was one of Petersdorf's favorites.

During medical school, Handsfield had considered various specialties—for a while, it was pediatrics, then hematology. When his internship ended, he stayed on in Seattle to do his residency in internal medicine. To Handsfield, Petersdorf personified internal medicine's reputation as the intellectual specialty.

"I've had three people that I can truly call mentors in my professional development," Handsfield said. "Petersdorf was the first."

The second was Marvin Turck.

"Marvin was the brightest know-the-details person I've ever known in medicine, and maybe anywhere, both in the lecture hall but especially on rounds," Handsfield said.

Turck and Petersdorf would riff off each other during case presentations. "Marvin was Petersdorf's protégé, but Marvin knew he was just as bright," Handsfield said. "They would sort of compete. They had a repartee."

Both Petersdorf and Turck used a standard gag line for particularly complex cases. They would go over possible diagnoses, then say, "Well, when all is said and done, your guess is as good as mine." Then, after a beat, add, "No, not as good as mine."

Turck, of course, had his stand-up routine of one-liners. "He was a nerdy guy by all the clichés," Handsfield said. "He wore his Jewishness on his sleeve with great pride. He was always telling Henny Youngman–type jokes. He was just incredibly fun to be around."

Handsfield had been able to defer his military obligation under the doctor draft until after he completed his training. As he wrapped up his residency, he began talking with Petersdorf and others about staying on to do an infectious-diseases fellowship. What interested him initially was to work on meningitis with Harry Beaty, himself a protégé of Petersdorf. But after talking to Beaty, Handsfield realized that he would be studying the disease mostly in laboratory animals.

So, in the informal manner in which fellowships were arranged in those days, Handsfield went to Turck and asked if he had any other options. "Marv in effect stole me from Harry," he said.

Handfield expected to start working with Turck on UTIs. Instead, when he showed up in Turck's office on the day his fellowship began, Turck asked, "Do you know King Holmes?"

And so Handsfield, although technically assigned to Turck, met his third mentor. That was when he learned he wouldn't be working on UTIs after all, though his reaction was different from Wiesner's. When Handsfield found out that Holmes's research focused on STIs, "That ratcheted up my interest even further," he said.

Partly it was the zeitgeist of the times. The 1967 "Summer of Love" had launched the free love movement. The popular press was full of stories about the sexual revolution.

But Handsfield's interest also was piqued by what Holmes knew that the news media was only starting to report: The new era brought skyrocketing rates of STDs, initially characterized as the "national gonorrhea epidemic"—and very little was known about them scientifically. He was intrigued by both Holmes's enthusiasm and his view on national public health and research priorities.

"It was an exciting new area to get into with a combination of interesting science, epidemiology, and social context," said Handsfield, who was King's fellow from 1971 to 1973. "If I'd stayed with Harry Beaty and meningitis, it wouldn't have had this new dynamic. This was truly the ground floor of what amounted to a whole new era."

Handsfield's early research followed two main tracks. In a three-year study started by Wiesner and Holmes among patients at UW hospitals, he identified and described 120 patients with disseminated gonococcal infection, or DGI—a kind of arthritis, often with skin rash, that occurs when gonorrhea bacteria enter the bloodstream. It remains the largest reported DGI case series.

That study led directly to his second research emphasis. Many men with DGI had genital (urethral) gonococcal infection without typical symptoms of gonorrhea. Although asymptomatic gonorrhea was known to be common in women, it was believed to be nearly nonexistent in men—yet here were all these cases. Working with Holmes and Jim Harnisch, Handsfield set out to study asymptomatic gonorrhea in men, including men without DGI, soon finding it to be far more common than previously believed.

That research revolutionized gonorrhea control and prevention. Men with gonorrhea had always been asked to refer their female partners for testing and treatment, knowing that many would be unknowingly infected. But it was thought unnecessary for infected women to refer their male partners because men would have symptoms and seek treatment on their own. The asymptomatic gonorrhea study—Handsfield's first[94] of several papers in the *New England Journal of Medicine*—demonstrated the importance of testing and treating all male partners of infected persons, regardless of symptoms. Handsfield's subsequent research neatly linked the two studies: it turned out that particular strains of gonorrhea are prone to cause both DGI and asymptomatic infection, and those strains were especially common in Seattle in the 1970s.

Handsfield was there at the beginning of Holmes's efforts to forge an academic–public health model that would eventually be adopted by STD programs throughout the country. Here and there, Handsfield said, academic programs and public health departments cooperated with one another, but generally they viewed each other across an oil-water divide. Universities saw county health departments as having no particular scientific expertise, especially in research. Health departments looked at universities as wanting access to patients as guinea pigs but lacking a commitment to the clinics' mission.

Holmes set out to bridge that divide. He started going by the Seattle–King County STD facility—then called the venereal disease clinic—to check the situation out. He found a staff that was overwhelmed by the sheer number of patients and who had only rudimentary training in providing health care of any kind. Nurses and others were staying long past the usual closing time to see everyone.

"It had been a clinic that you could usually close up and go home at 4:00 p.m.," Holmes said, recalling his first visit there. "But it was packed with people because there was an epidemic of STDs of various sorts."[95]

He saw an opportunity. Would it be helpful, he asked, if the university were to staff a second clinic with hours starting at 4:00 p.m.? Alf Pedersen, the clinic director and an accomplished clinician and epidemiologist, almost shouted: "Yes!"

"You never saw such happy people in your life," Holmes said. "That's how we set up the collaboration, as simple as that."

Holmes only made it look simple. Setting up what would become known worldwide as the "Seattle model" of cooperation between academic research centers and public health clinics meant not just working out logistics but building relationships. Crucially, it also meant dramatically improving clinical training, followed in a few years by vastly improved clinical skills as a condition of employment.

The new STD clinic opened at Harborview Medical Center—owned by King County and operated by the university—on Valentine's day 1972, with Holmes as its founding director. Soon, he and his two young fellows, Wiesner and Handsfield, had a third fellow to help with evening shifts and research projects.

The dermatologist: James Harnisch

A Notre Dame graduate who had been a guard on the Fighting Irish football team, Jim Harnisch, a year younger than Handsfield, received his medical degree from Ohio State University in 1969. He did his residency in internal medicine at Grady Memorial Hospital in Atlanta where, decades earlier, Paul Beeson had held rounds as chair of medicine at Emory School of Medicine.

Grady is one of the largest and busiest public hospitals in the country, and residencies there were known for being especially challenging. Harnisch was on duty every other night for two years. As is common at many public hospitals, the patients he treated were among the poorest of the poor, without health insurance or access to regular health care. The experience of caring for—and earning the trust of—a largely underserved, and often stigmatized, population prepared him for the work he would later do in Seattle.

While at Grady, he tried to do research on top of his heavy clinical load, putting in laboratory time to work on a meningitis study using rabbits. He was interested in both infectious diseases and dermatology, once encountering a patient he suspected of having leprosy. It turned out that the mysterious ulcerations on the patient's feet were due to diabetes, but it sparked a lifelong interest in Hansen's disease that would continue in Seattle.

What brought him to Seattle was, indirectly, the doctor draft. When his residency ended, Harnisch sought to fulfill his military requirement by joining the CDC's EIS. Already highly selective, it had become an even more sought-after appointment as the Vietnam War escalated.[96] The EIS offered him a position, but it would not start until the following year—too late. However, the CDC Venereal Diseases Division[97] had an immediate opening and it also met his military obligation. He took it.

Just three weeks after his training began, he met King Holmes at a conference in Atlanta. Holmes made an instant impression.

"From the questions he asked, it was clear that he had a very probing mind," Harnisch said. "He wanted to advance our understanding of sexually transmitted diseases. I realized this was a bright man whose goals I shared and who was going to be very productive in medicine."[98]

When the CDC offered Harnisch his choice of a posting in Memphis, San Francisco, or Seattle, Harnisch didn't hesitate. He chose Seattle because Holmes was there.

He was assigned to the Seattle–King County Public Health Department's VD Clinic. He arrived just as Holmes was setting up the collaboration between the university and the health department for a second, academically run evening STD clinic at Harborview.

"After Dr. Holmes got used to me," Harnisch said, "he basically offered me an infectious diseases fellowship while I was doing my CDC responsibility." Just as Marvin Turck had become Petersdorf's fellow while working for the EIS, Harnisch began doing double duty as Holmes's fellow and as a CDC officer.

Holmes recalled one of their early projects as especially memorable.

"We had this huge outbreak of people coming in, male and female. It turned out they were part of a swingers' club," he said. "That's where Jim got started."[99]

The Seattle area, it turned out, had a vibrant swingers' scene. There were swingers who lived in Seattle and swingers who lived across Lake Washington in Bellevue. One club was made up of motorcycle swingers. What they shared in common was sex—lots of it, with as many partners as possible in an evening.

A couple from one of the clubs came to the county clinic to ask what to do about an outbreak of gonorrhea in the group, which numbered about 60 or 70. Previously, clinicians had treated individual infections and urged the club's members to use condoms. But no one did, and the outbreak continued.

Harnisch came up with the idea of testing all the members of the group and, if their tests were normal, giving them a card that said: "Approved for sex by Dr. H." They were instructed to exchange cards before they had sex.

He recalled Handsfield saying at the time, "I can't believe you did that! Do you realize they're having sex over your name?"

Harnisch was unperturbed. "We finally stamped out gonorrhea in this group," he said. He and Holmes wrote up a paper on the outbreak. "It wasn't 'Hey, this is practice-changing," Harnisch said. "More, 'Hey, this is interesting.'"

But the journals weren't interested. The Interscience Conference on Antimicrobial Agents and Chemotherapy, or ICAAC, the main infectious-diseases conference of the day, also rejected their proposal to present the case—which they had titled "GC Swings," using the acronym for gonococcal disease.

Holmes conceded that the title was "rather irreverent," but added, "It would have been the most popular presentation at that particular meeting."

It was hardly the only tongue-in-cheek title. Earlier, Handsfield had written a case report of a single male with gonorrhea who had infected at least seven women. Handsfield and Holmes had called the man "GC," for both the gonococcus bacteria and for "Gonorrhea Charlie," as in Typhoid Mary. (It didn't fly either.) In 1976, Holmes cowrote, with Jennifer Wear, a guide for the general public on STIs called *How to Have Intercourse Without Getting Screwed*.

The irreverence challenged the prevailing attitude. In those years most other infectious-diseases researchers still looked down on STD research. Many people—including health professionals—were uncomfortable talking or hearing about sexuality, much less STDs. But the young UW infectious-diseases researchers, almost all in their 20s or early 30s, were part of a generation in transition. Their parents did not talk about sex, but their peers did. They came of age as the women's and gay rights movements were changing sexual practices.

"We were from a youthful generation that was more comfortable with sex and sexuality and all that went with it, both in terms of how we dealt with patients and what we learned from patients and the research that we were immersed in," Handsfield said. "It was part and parcel of the fun of it."

For researchers who were straight, part of the learning curve was understanding sexual practices of gay men. That sometimes involved awkward moments.

Soon after Harnisch's arrival, he joined Holmes and Wiesner in research to understand the frequency of gonorrhea in men who have sex with men. The project involved collecting swabs and testing men for gonorrhea at all possibly exposed anatomic sites. The best way to get a lot of samples quickly was to go to where lots of gay men met for sex. Handsfield joined in for some of the testing sessions.

One night the four researchers paid admission to a late-night dance party at a gay bathhouse near downtown Seattle's Pioneer Square. They set up a makeshift clinic in the back with small screens to provide some privacy, and if patrons agreed to be part of the research project, they were swabbed and tested then and there. From behind the screens one or the other researchers could be heard saying to volunteers, "OK, bend over. Now hold them apart. Perfect—this'll be quick!"

This was all new, and at this early time in their research careers, the four were not immune to some natural anxiety—perhaps especially the former Notre Dame student. Suddenly, the power failed, all the lights went out, and the already dimly lit room turned pitch black. About four seconds of silence passed. Then Harnisch, sounding every bit the Fighting Irish football guard, boomed out, "Nobody move!"

He quickly followed with, "Don't worry, everybody! Everything's OK!"

Being a straight man working with gay men during those times involved earning their trust, Harnisch said years later, much as he had earned the trust of the often-stigmatized communities he worked with at Grady Memorial in Atlanta.

"As long as we demonstrated that we actually cared about them and their health, they sensed it," he said.

Still, there was that learning curve. Harnisch always tried to avoid scientific jargon in his community talks and to use terms his patients used. From his work with men, he'd grown accustomed to saying "balling" or "screwing." When a lesbian group called to ask him to give a talk about gay women and STDs, he used those terms in his talk to the dozens of women who had gathered. Afterward, one of them came up to him and said, "Dr. Harnisch, thank you for coming. We enjoyed your talk. Except we don't ball or screw."

"I turned red," said Harnisch. "I thought, 'Oh, boy.'"

Irreverent humor was one way to get through the awkwardness. A neighbor known for being a gossip once said to Harnisch's wife, Kathy, "I haven't seen Jim around much." Kathy Harnisch, who shared her husband's dry wit, replied, "He's resting because he has to go to a gay dance tonight." As she knew would happen, the neighbor turned and almost ran back to the house, so eager was she to start calling people in the neighborhood with the news.

Working on STDs may not—at first—have carried the same status as working on other infections. But that was changing. Holmes and his growing team were producing research findings that journals could no longer ignore.

Harnisch and Holmes published one of the first papers to show high rates of STDs in men who have sex with men and also the high incidence of hepatitis B among the male gay population, which had not been shown before. Handsfield, Harnisch, and Holmes reported that gonorrhea could be asymptomatic in men, upending the accepted orthodoxy and leading to revised guidelines for partner notifications. Paul Wiesner did one of the first studies to look at the frequency of non-genital gonorrhea in men who had sex with men. It was known by anyone studying STDs that gay men had both anal and oral sex and that infections could occur in sites other than the genitals, but no one had done systematic research to know how frequently such infections occurred or how to treat them.

"Every month, by publishing a new *New England Journal of Medicine* paper, King would keep ratcheting up the bar," said David Eschenbach, another of Holmes's early fellows. "All of a sudden, by three or four years, researching sexually transmitted diseases were seen as equal to people who studied urinary tract infections, like Marv Turck, or pneumonia. And it was solely because of King's work."

The obstetrician-gynecologist: David Eschenbach

David Eschenbach received his medical degree from the University of Wisconsin in 1968. He arrived in Seattle as part of the last group to do rotating internships—that is, to spend the first year after medical school rotating through internal medicine, surgery, orthopedics, and obstetrics and gynecology—before starting his residency in obstetrics and gynecology.

By the time Eschenbach got to his final year of residency in 1972, he felt that he had already mastered a lot of what he needed to know to practice his specialty. So he asked his OB-GYN department chairman, Walter Herman, about undertaking a research project. Herman mentioned the request to his good friend, the chairman of the Department of Medicine, Robert Petersdorf.

"Petersdorf was one of those people who thought outside the box," said Eschenbach.[100] His out-of-the-box idea was to have the OB-GYN resident work with Holmes on genital infections.

Holmes welcomed the cross-fertilization. According to Eschenbach, he also liked that Eschenbach's modest salary would be paid through a Ford Foundation grant of Herman's.

Eschenbach's project was to investigate which organisms caused PID, a serious complication of STIs in women that could lead to chronic pelvic pain, infertility, and life-threatening ectopic pregnancies. The syndrome was believed to be caused by gonorrhea, but Holmes was interested in knowing whether—like the infections he had seen in men in the Western Pacific while in the Navy—there were additional microbes in play.

Carrying out the research meant late hours for Eschenbach. Women tended to feel painful symptoms of infection late in the day, often realizing by 11:00 p.m. or midnight that they were not going to be able to get to sleep. That's when they would start drifting into the emergency room. That's when Eschenbach needed to be there.

"I'm there from midnight until 4 in the morning, doing all of these interviews and sampling the cervix and the vagina," he said. "We actually put needles in through the lower part of the vagina—you can go in through the abdominal cavity and suck out pus. I would plate them out in the middle of the night and put them in special jars, so they weren't exposed to the air, and we'd have a microbiologist look at these results."

Having grown up on a Wisconsin dairy farm where rising at dawn and working 14-hour days was normal, Eschenbach was a good fit for the long hours. Spending all night in the ER "was pretty easy work" compared to the farm, he said.

Besides, being called in the middle of the night or on weekends to deliver babies was standard practice for an obstetrician.

"I was driven to do it, and King was supportive of it," he said of the project. "We'd put in enough cool things to make it interesting. It was my idea to get the pus out of the abdomen, and it was his idea to associate with an anerobic microbiologist—that was something that hadn't been done before."

Over six months, Eschenbach interviewed and took samples from around 100 patients at all three UW teaching hospitals—the Public Health Service Hospital, Harborview, and the UW Medical Center. In 1974, his residency completed, he returned to train formally with King as an ID fellow, an unusual move for an OB-GYN. He picked up the research project again and interviewed another 100 patients for a total of 204.

Harnisch and others pitched in. Harnisch recalled how, if he iden-tified a woman with PID while working at the health department, he would ask her if she would like to take part in a research project that would in turn provide free care.

"Once she agreed," he said, "I would call David Eschenbach, and he would drive up to the Public Health building. I would walk the woman out, open the car door, put her in his car, and he would drive her to the hospital. That's how basic our study was—the physician drove the patient to the hospital."

If collecting the samples was hard work, working with Holmes to put a paper together was almost as grueling.

"You would wait an hour or two because he was always behind, yet when you were in that room, the concentration was on you and your project," Eschenbach said. "And it *was* concentrated."

First came the thinking-through of the study design and then the thinking-through of the results. Holmes had begun editing a textbook on infectious diseases, and he'd hired Wiesner and others to help. But he would still go over every single word himself. So the breadth of knowledge—on the epidemiology, the molecular biology, the behavioral psychology of STDs—he could bring to a research project was astounding.

"He would look at it in a different way and present it in a way that was different from what you'd originally intended," Eschenbach said. "He was incredibly diverse and bright and just into everything. He would come off the wall with the craziest ideas, and I would fight him on them. And every time he was right."

Then there was the actual writing. That, too, could be a painful process. Holmes went over the paper not just line by line but word for word—in virtually indecipherable handwriting. Eschenbach often had to write 10 or 12 drafts before Holmes was satisfied.

But the reward was worth it. Eschenbach had grown up in a German community with a grandfather who still spoke the language, and working with Holmes, he came to realize that his own sentence structure was more German than English.

"Anybody else would have just given up and said, 'It's a mess,'" he said of his early drafts. Not Holmes. He continued to work with Eschenbach in his calm way, line by line and word by word.

The reward was more than publication in top journals.

"I got tears in my eyes a couple of times after I presented at a conference," Eschenbach said. "People would come up to me and say,

'I really enjoyed your presentation. It was so well written.' I'd think, 'You have no idea how many hours I've sweated over this.'"

Eschenbach may have thought the revisions were due to his German background, but everybody has a story to tell about Holmes as an editor. Back in 1971, Wiesner had warned Handsfield "Don't work too hard on your first draft for King. He'll make just as many changes whether you've spent two hours or twenty." Handsfield didn't listen. Believing himself to be a pretty good writer, he was initially pleased that the first draft of his first paper came back without a mark. Then Holmes asked, "What was your verbal SAT score?" After Handsfield told him, Holmes said, "You can do better than this. Start over."

Harnisch's record was 15 revisions. "He would meet with you at any point in time if you were writing a paper," Harnisch said. "He would meet with me at 8 or 10 at night or on Sunday mornings."

And yet, for someone so intense, Holmes was also remarkably relaxed—which made 15 revisions tolerable.

"He almost never got super excited or angry," Harnisch said.

Eschenbach agreed. "He has a Type A personality, but he's also totally calm," he said. "When you talk with him, he'll ask what you're doing in a very nice, conversational way. But then you realize afterward, 'I just got interviewed.' So his personality is really low-key, but it's intense."

Eschenbach's research, published in the *New England Journal of Medicine*,[101] for the first time focused on the role of anaerobic infections in PID and helped set up a treatment trial that he did with the CDC. It remains a seminal paper on the polymicrobial etiology of PID—in part because of the difficulty in repeating a project that involved testing more than 200 women, without prior notice, in the middle of the night.

Among Eschenbach's other early accomplishments was the discovery, with Holmes, that the Dalkon Shield IUD caused PID, leading to the device being taken off the market. He would go on to help create a subspecialty in OB-GYN infectious diseases. He also chaired UW's ob-gyn department for 16 years, keeping his hand in research, especially the role of infections in premature births. He continued to collaborate periodically with Holmes.

"King's got a way of learning about what you're doing, and he brings you back in, even 30 years out," he said. "There is probably no better mentor at the university. He always looks after you."

Harnisch, who followed in Holmes's footsteps to become Turck's chief resident, went on to train in his other passion, dermatology. He would split his time between private and public practice, but he too would be called back by King in later years—to set up a leprosy clinic.

Handsfield, Harnisch, and Eschenbach would each play a key role in building and expanding the influence of Seattle and the University of Washington in infectious-diseases research and practice.

A fourth fellow, Walter W. Karney, a US Navy captain, went on to become a professor at the Uniformed Services University of the Health Sciences in Bethesda, Maryland. Although Karney did not continue to focus primarily on STD research, he facilitated other UW researchers' work with the Navy and later served as manager of the Navy HIV program of the US Naval Medical Command.[102]

And King's first fellow, Paul Wiesner, left Seattle in 1972, immediately after his fellowship ended, to enter the US Public Health Service at the Center for Disease Control[103] in Atlanta, where he was named director of the Division of Sexually Transmitted Diseases. The ex-seminarian became the nation's top public health official for STDs.

Beyond STDs

The impact of Holmes and his fellows on the field was swift. In the early 1970s, the main scientific meeting for infectious diseases, the Interscience Conference on Antimicrobial Agents and Chemotherapy, or ICAAC (universally pronounced "ick-ack") for the first time held a scientific abstract session for oral research presentations devoted entirely to STDs. Of eight papers presented, six were from the UW—all coauthored by King and presented by him or his fellows.

But not everything in their fellowship years focused entirely on STDs. Harnisch worked with Turck and King in 1972 to investigate a large outbreak of cutaneous diphtheria in Seattle's Skid Road area near Pioneer Square. (Harnisch had a standing battle with Robert Petersdorf over the correct name for this area; Petersdorf would change his text to say "skid row" and Harnisch would change it back. "Skid row" as a euphemism for lower-class work environments originated in Seattle's pioneer days, when loggers had—literally—created roads by skidding timber downhill to Puget Sound.)

The cutaneous diphtheria outbreak occurred among people who were both homeless and alcoholics. Many of them would wind up in jail, and since Harnisch and Handsfield worked as jail physicians on Friday nights, they were able to get cultures to test for diphtheria. The problem was tracking down folks who tested positive for treatment once they got out of jail, since no one had an address.

Harnisch got creative in his search. He told the Seattle police chief that the outbreak was a health emergency, albeit not an officially designated one, so the chief assigned him two police officers and a paddy wagon. Wearing a black raincoat and flashing his CDC badge, Harnisch went to Pioneer Square bars to look for those who needed treatment. The bartender would nod and give a jerk of his chin to point out the missing patient. The two officers would load up the paddy wagon and Harnisch would deliver the patients to Seattle's repurposed TB hospital, where they were given antitoxin along with seven days of antibiotics to cure their diphtheria and then were discharged.

But the real solution came after Harnisch and Holmes—following Holmes's dictum from the West Pacific to go into the field—went to have a look at the drunk tank. At that time, police would arrest and jail anyone who was drunk in public or just wandering the streets and hold them in two large jailed areas at the police station, hence the term drunk tank.

"It was awful," Holmes said. "People were lying on top of each other." In the crowded, unsanitary conditions, the skin infections spread easily.

"So we got them to do away with the drunk tank, and diphtheria went away," Holmes said.[104]

Meanwhile, Petersdorf, despite his heavy administrative duties, also managed to keep a hand in research dealing with fever, meningitis, antibiotic pharmacology and—in collaboration with Turck—UTIs. But he felt that he was working more and more through surrogates. So in 1971, he took a sabbatical to England to focus on research again with Paul Beeson.

Beeson was at that time the Nuffield professor of medicine at Oxford, having surprised everyone by going back to the laboratory after 13 years as chair of medicine at Yale. Petersdorf took advantage of Beeson's "remarkable gift for asking the right clinical questions"[105] and spent his sabbatical investigating endocarditis, an interest he would follow for the rest of his career.

"During my year at Oxford, Beeson rejuvenated my investigative career," Petersdorf wrote. "My contact with endocarditis began in Oxford in 1971 and has continued ever since."

He also undertook another project: recruiting Beeson to Seattle. When Beeson left Oxford to return to the United States in 1974, he became a Veterans' Administration Distinguished Professor of Medicine at the Seattle VA Medical Center, affiliated with the University of Washington, his undergraduate alma mater.

Upon his arrival, Beeson sought out Harnisch to learn about his diphtheria research, telling Harnisch about his father's experience delivering antitoxin via dog sled to a suspected diphtheria patient in rural Alaska. Harnisch grew close to Beeson and became his family's physician. "He was one of the giants of medicine," Harnisch said.

He was not the only one.

"We had some real giants here, with Beeson and Petersdorf and with people like Marv and King," said Eschenbach. "Seattle was *the* place for infectious diseases."

5

Atlanta
to Seattle

They met in Atlanta at the start of their careers—three young disease-detectives-in-training in the EIS. Walter E. Stamm, Lawrence Corey, and Joel D. Meyers forged friendships there that deepened in Seattle, where they made lives, careers, and their mark on infectious-diseases research worldwide.

Born in Philadelphia in 1945, Walt Stamm grew up in Portland, Oregon. He had a golden boy quality, and it wasn't just his West Coast upbringing. In high school, he was student body president, excelled in football, basketball and baseball, *and* graduated at the top of his class. And so it went throughout his life.

In college at Stanford, where he also shone in both sports and academics, he met another Portlandian, Peggy Carstensen. They married a semester after he started Harvard Medical School and then returned to the Pacific Northwest for his residency at the University of Washington. David C. Dale, the chief resident at the UW Medical Center when Stamm arrived, liked him instantly—as did everyone. "He was kind, considerate, loyal and just plain smart," Dale wrote.[106]

After his residency, Stamm joined the EIS and was assigned to the coveted hospital infections branch, where he rose to be chief. Among the notable investigations he led was one into an outbreak of UTIs among patients in a hospital in New Jersey; it helped define the role that invasive devices such as catheters can play in producing life-threatening infections.

Early on, about four months into his tour of duty, he was sent to work up an outbreak of hepatitis in a hemodialysis unit in Valhalla, New York. Accompanying him was another newly minted EIS officer, Larry Corey. The collaboration launched a lifelong friendship between two men of such different backgrounds and temperaments that Corey would call them the academic odd couple.

Two years younger than Stamm and Meyers, Corey grew up with two older sisters in Detroit, the children of immigrants from Russia and Poland. His father was in the *schmatte*, or rag recycling, business well before recycling became profitable; his mother was a homemaker. Corey was the "Americanized one" who would later kick himself for not learning the Yiddish, Russian, Polish, Ukrainian, and Hebrew languages that filled his household.

He decided on a career in medicine at age 10 when his oldest sister married a man who was training to be an ophthalmologist. The choice was sealed when his other sister also married a physician. Collecting scholarships and skipping grades, Corey graduated from the University of Michigan at 20 to enter the university's fast-tracked, three-year medical program. Along the way, he met and married Amy Glasser, whose father had supervised the field trials of the Salk polio vaccine. Dr. Jonas Salk was a guest at their 1969 wedding.

When he met one of the great vaccine developers in history, Corey was leaning toward a career in cardiology, not infectious diseases. In medical school, he and two like-minded friends had even led a walkout of a public health class taught by another pioneering vaccine developer, virologist and epidemiologist Tommy Francis, who was Salk's mentor. Francis was the first to isolate the influenza B virus and developed early flu vaccines during World War II, but the students maintained that he was not teaching them what they needed to know about health care in today's world.

Corey and his classmates pressed for a greater voice in what and how they were taught. With two others, he collected their arguments into a book, called "Medicine in a Changing Society," which was published in 1972 with contributions from notable health reformers such as Massachusetts Senator Edward M. Kennedy. "In today's society," the three students wrote in its preface, "it is not possible to be an effective physician without understanding the social issues and moral, ethical, and organized problems that derive from the setting in which medicine is practiced."[107]

The work showed an early academic bent as well as an interest in the kind of policymaking and community engagement Corey would come to practice. It also showed more than a bit of youthful hubris, as he would realize when he landed in the EIS. Assigned to the viral diseases division, he reread—and newly appreciated—Tommy Francis's papers on influenza.

"It was one of life's great ironies," he said. "It was instructive. And in retrospect sort of funny."[108]

But before Atlanta, while he was doing his residency at the University of Michigan, a family crisis struck: The brother-in-law Corey idolized—who had first inspired him to enter medicine—was diagnosed with Hodgkin lymphoma. His sister accompanied her husband to Stanford for treatment while the Coreys took care of their children, with Corey commuting into Ann Arbor to finish his training.

The draft was looming when Corey heard about the EIS through a former medical school classmate. He would later say that Stamm joined the EIS "because he trained at the University of Washington, where infectious disease was a dominant intellectual focus of the Department of Medicine and he was interested in ID. I went there because my draft number was 4 and I needed an option out of Vietnam."[109]

Once in Atlanta, the work on viral diseases began to intrigue him.

The EIS was one of the premier places in the world to learn to investigate disease outbreaks, but years later Corey described his and Stamm's early assignment with characteristic dry humor.

"We were classic EIS guys—experts defined as someone with a box of slides and more than 100 miles from home," he said. "Walt solved the mystery of the outbreak and I knew the name of the bug. So, we wrote my first and his second *New England Journal of Medicine* paper on this together."[110]

The best outcome, he would later say, was his and Amy's lifelong friendship with Walt and Peggy Stamm. They had children the same age. They played tennis together and started a dinner club that continued in Seattle. And increasingly, Corey and Stamm bonded over the intellectual challenges of the work they were doing.

Then, on Christmas day, barely six months after Corey arrived in Atlanta, his brother-in-law died. The harsh therapy had vanquished his cancer but so weakened his immune system that he died of an infection. He was 37, Corey, 26.

"You could say I've never recovered from that," Corey said. "He was like my brother."[111]

His work in infectious diseases took on new meaning. He did his first vaccine study on influenza with Walter Dowdle, whose work for the CDC helped lay the scientific foundation for successful prevention campaigns for flu, hepatitis, and polio and, years later, provided the foundation for Corey's interest in herpes and HIV vaccines. Drawing on lessons learned from Francis and Salk, Corey wrote articles on influenza for the CDC's influential Morbidity and Mortality Weekly Report (MMWR). MMWR editor Michael Greg red-lined every page, honing the skills Corey had learned from his 10th grade English teacher and preparing him for later encounters with King Holmes's infamous red pen.

Amy Corey would join him at their dining room table, her tidier handwriting keeping the line listings of patients enrolled in studies legible. He investigated a hepatis outbreak in Atlanta, published articles on the treatment and prevention of rabies, and did some of the early investigations of Reye's syndrome, a rare but sometimes deadly swelling of the brain and liver in children and teenagers recovering from viral illnesses. He reported on cases of influenza B–associated Reye's syndrome in a county in Michigan, discussed the likelihood of lowering the incidence by vaccinating children against influenza B, and supported the hypothesis that the use of aspirin was associated with the disease. (Subsequent investigations continued to demonstrate this association, and reducing aspirin use in children with influenza has been associated with disappearance of the syndrome.)

Seeing Corey's growing interest, Stamm suggested that he consider the University of Washington for further training in infectious diseases when his EIS stint was over. At a meeting with Marvin Turck in Chicago at the Interscience Conference on Antimicrobial Agents and Chemotherapy, Corey found himself recruited to do just that.

Stamm stayed on in Atlanta for a third year with the EIS before returning to Seattle himself to be chief resident at Harborview. Corey arrived a year before him, in 1975, along with another good friend from the EIS: Joel Meyers.

Born in Detroit in 1945, Meyers graduated with honors from Dartmouth College and Harvard Medical School, then did his internship and one year of residency in internal medicine at the University of Pennsylvania. He moved to Atlanta in 1972—the year before Corey and Stamm—to fulfill his military obligation through the EIS.

Meyers was extraordinarily bright yet self-effacing, with a wry little smile and a wicked wit. On a blind date, he met his future wife—Barbara Thrasher, a teacher who was also new to Atlanta. From the moment they met, Thrasher said she had "this overwhelming feeling that this is the person."[112] Meyers and Thrasher later became friends with the Coreys and Stamms, adding their sparkle and charm to gatherings and ski trips.

During his time in Atlanta, Meyers made another pivotal connection, one that would determine the course of his career and help establish a new research area in the field of infectious diseases. The EIS sent him on assignment to Seattle, where Don Thomas was continuing his work on bone marrow transplantation. Dispatched to investigate an outbreak of what turned out to be hepatitis C among Thomas's immune-compromised patients, Meyers traced the source of the outbreak to platelet and plasma donation and platelet transfusion.

"Joel's work on this outbreak," Corey said, "really illustrated the importance that the discipline of infectious disease had for the marrow transplant patient."[113]

Meyers described the investigation in a paper jointly authored with Thomas and King Holmes, the first of several Meyers would write over the years on the same outbreak as scientists identified a new type of hepatitis and developed new screening tests, and he was able to retest stored samples. He also fell in love with Seattle and with the team doing such cutting-edge transplantation work.

When his EIS stint ended, Meyers returned to Pennsylvania to finish his residency. But his perseverance and skill had impressed the hard-to-impress Thomas, who lobbied for Meyers to come back to Seattle. Meyers did, first as an infectious-diseases fellow and then to head a brand-new program investigating infections that plague immune-compromised patients.

He and Thrasher loaded up their car and drove from Pennsylvania. They arrived in Seattle on a sparkling day in June 1975. Sailboats dotted Lake Washington, and Mount Rainier dominated the horizon.

"Do people actually get to live like this?" Thrasher remembered thinking. "We'd never seen anything like that in the East."[114]

The land of giants

Corey had never seen anything like Seattle either. The rugged beauty of the Pacific Northwest was a physical manifestation of the "incredible sort of West Coast freedom" he found in a division that was still being invented.

"It was like, OK, it's beautiful out here, and you were supposed to be this individualistic person and go out and build your own program," he said. "If you're feeling depressed, you can go out and chop wood or take a hike."

The UW School of Medicine was launched during an era of enthusiasm for medical research and abundant government funding. In the post–World War II boom years, the NIH was so flush with cash that the running joke among biomedical researchers of every specialty was, "While you're up, get me another grant."

UW researchers were up a lot.

Petersdorf was busy building a powerhouse Department of Medicine. He also kept a hand in his own endocarditis research begun during his sabbatical with Beeson, published papers and edited a textbook, and held leadership positions in virtually every key medical association. But he still made time to hold rounds—sometimes from the edge of the university pool, where he swam laps every noon hour— bluntly demanding the best from students and trainees and, as always, keeping his eye out for exceptional talent.

Bill Kirby had stepped away from administering the infectious- diseases division to devote more time to his research testing the new antibiotics still being developed, but he remained very much involved in training and was revered by students and trainees. Every day, the clinical microbiology lab held an hour-long session called plate rounds, over which he presided. A train of students, residents, and fellows would arrive in the lab to look at auger plates and discuss which bacteria were growing on them.

Kirby was phenomenally good at plate rounds. He had a "stunning breadth of knowledge about all microorganisms that might be cultured from the human body," according to Stanley Falkow, a celebrated microbial geneticist who had been drawn to the UW in 1972 by Kirby, Petersdorf, and John Sherris, by then chair of microbiology. "I always thought that plate rounds provided me with a unique view of the natural history of microorganisms that inhabit humans," Falkow said, "akin to what Darwin did while he wandered the Galapagos looking at finches."[115]

Seymour Klebanoff had taken over as head of the ID division in 1974, and Marvin Turck was chief of medicine at the Public Health Service Hospital. Paul Beeson was an eminent white-haired presence at the VA hospital, regaling fellows with his breadth of knowledge at monthly infectious-diseases dinners.

"In our field, except for Maxwell Finland and one or two people in Boston, the most successful people were here," Corey said, recalling the faculty in place when he arrived at the UW. "This program was one of the centers of the universe."

Like Handsfield before him, Corey thought he would be working with Turck. But, also like Handsfield, he found out after he arrived that his mentor would be King Holmes.

Holmes had secured a training grant from the NIH, one of the first the NIH awarded in what was still called venereal diseases. The NIH was surprised to receive an application from such a junior faculty member, so the head of the National Institute of Allergies and Infectious Diseases traveled to Seattle to check Holmes out. Anticipating that reaction, Holmes had rounded up a stellar group of senior faculty members from across departments willing to serve as mentors. Among them were two from the newly formed UW School of Public Health—George Kenny, chair of the Department of Pathobiology, and E. Russell Alexander, chair of the Department of Epidemiology.

Kenny had joined what was then UW's Department of Preventive Medicine in 1961 with a PhD in microbiology from the University of Minnesota. He was known for research on mycoplasmas, organisms that cause "walking pneumonia." Alexander came to the UW in 1960 from Atlanta, yet another veteran of the famed EIS. A big teddy bear of a man with a laser-like mind, he was an internationally respected epidemiologist and pediatric infectious-diseases specialist.

Holmes also recruited Falkow, who was revolutionizing microbiology by using genetics to better understand how infecting microbes interact with host cells to cause disease. In work at the UW and later at Stanford, Falkow showed how antibiotic resistance spreads from one bacterium to another via tiny DNA rings known as plasmids and how plasmids can also transfer toxins that turn once-harmless microbes deadly. King described him as "probably the smartest guy we ever had."

Seeing such expertise on board, the NIH approved Holmes's training grant application—and continued to renew it for five decades. By then Holmes had moved his trainees out of the giant restroom and into trailers on the Public Health Service Hospital grounds. He was expanding not just his research program and the number of trainees but the field of STDs itself.

At the time Holmes started, gonorrhea and syphilis were the two best known of the six infections considered venereal diseases. But Holmes, and soon a cadre of fellows and former fellows were working to explore new pathogens and find better ways to diagnose, treat, and prevent them. Over his five decades of research, the number of pathogens known to be sexually transmitted rose from 6 to 35; at least 20 were studied by Holmes or his fellows.

Corey would become an international expert on one of the emerging pathogens. But he didn't know that at the time of his first lunch with Holmes in the cafeteria of the PHS Hospital. Holmes asked the requisite, "Tell me about yourself," and Corey, having worked on flu and hepatitis at the EIS, replied that he was interested in viral diseases.

Holmes looked at him and said, in his calm, understated way, "Well, I'm interested in sex."

There was, Holmes continued, a lifelong, recurring viral infection called genital herpes that had no treatment and that no one really knew much about. Would Corey be interested in pursuing it?

Corey turned almost as pale as Paul Wiesner had.

"Kosher home, grandfather's a rabbi in the old country ... studious ... basically a nerd ... and then going to work on sexually transmitted diseases," he wrote years later for a 1988 lecture on receiving an award for work in precisely that area. "My mother was telling people I was going to be a cardiologist. What was I doing here!!"[116]

Recalling that conversation, Holmes said, "I thought I'd lost him."[117]

He had not.

Off they went

The UW was not, Corey found, the kind of place where you worked for your mentor. It was a place where your mentor sort of gave you an idea and basically said, "Off you go!"

What happened next Corey attributed to luck, but he was ready—and driven—to make good use of it. Very early in his fellowship, a "marvelous drug dropped into my lap," as he put it. He led the clinical trials that took the drug from the bench to the bedside.

The drug was acyclovir. Developed by biochemist Gertrude Elion at Burroughs Wellcome (now GlaxoSmithKline), it was a new type of drug directed for the first time at an enzyme specific for a virus—in this case, the herpesvirus—to control and suppress a viral infection.

King set up the first meeting with Elion, and Corey came away enamored with what she was doing.

Elion was in her 60s when Corey started working with her, making multiple trips to North Carolina's Research Triangle Park. She had numerous drug successes behind her and was well on her way to the Nobel Prize she would share with George Hitchings in 1988.

"She took me under her wing," he said. "It was really great fun just listening to her—learning what laboratory science was, how to investigate things, just the clarity of her thinking and how nice she was."

He designed a clinical trial of a topical version of acyclovir. It was not a cure, but it showed that the treatment was safe and led to a published paper and more funding. Corey pressed on, hiring a nurse, Carol Winter, and running a clinic on the second floor of Harborview Medical Center. "We were, and still are, the only research clinic devoted entirely to herpes," he said.

Business was booming. The sexual revolution that had crowded the Seattle–King County venereal diseases clinic packed Corey's herpes clinic. In a few years, *Time* magazine would famously feature herpes on its cover with the caption, "Today's Scarlet Letter,"[118] foreshadowing the even greater fear and stigma that would come with AIDS.

Corey continued to work with Elion through his fellowship and as a young faculty member. The breakthrough came in a randomized trial of acyclovir delivered by IV to 17 women with severe genital herpes.

Going forward on the trial was nerve-wracking. Half the scientists Corey knew not only doubted that an antiviral would work, they feared it would cause harm, attacking human cells rather than the virus and causing an autoimmune disorder or even cancer.

But Elion assured him otherwise. "Wait a minute, Larry," he recalled her telling him. "This drug recognizes an enzyme that only the virus makes. Have confidence. I don't think it's going to cause any problems."

"She gave me confidence that the drug would work," Corey said. "I was young enough and bold enough to say, 'Let's see what this drug can do.'"

It was clear within 48 hours that the drug was working to—for the first time—control and suppress a viral infection. Results were so striking that Corey could tell who was getting the therapy and who the placebo, even though neither the researchers nor the patients in the double-blinded study knew. Corey remembers exchanging a look with Carol Winter. Each was thinking, "Wow, there's something special going on here."

Joel Meyers also worked with Elion. He tested acyclovir in bone marrow transplant patients whose immune systems had been destroyed by treatment and pretransplant conditioning, allowing once-latent herpesvirus infections to reactivate and cause severe complications not seen in healthy people. Corey, still grieving his brother-in-law's death, was relieved that Meyers ran these trials. Treating cancer patients would have been too painful a reminder.

Meyers, too, saw dramatic results. He brought photographs to show Elion of young adults recovering from bone marrow transplants, their infections safely treated. Elion would relish hearing his and Corey's stories of how patients responded.

Next up was developing and testing an oral version of the drug. The principles behind acyclovir would later lead to the development of the AIDS drug AZT and to treatments for hepatitis B and hepatitis C.

"Acyclovir changed everything," Corey said. "First King changed everything in recognizing that there were sexually transmitted viruses. And the first important sexually transmitted virus was genital herpes. So I was working on the first one, and we had the first antiviral. Then we started this whole world of treating transplantation infections."

Meyers never really had an ID mentor. He worked mainly with Don Thomas and the oncologists on the bone marrow transplantation team.

By then the team had moved to the newly founded Fred Hutchinson Cancer Research Center, where Thomas was director of medical oncology.

"Dr. Thomas recognized the importance of recruiting different specialists to improve transplantation on multiple fronts," recalled Rainer Storb, a bone marrow transplant pioneer who began working with Thomas in 1965. Thomas recruited Meyers, Storb said, "who laid the groundwork for what is now the largest group of infectious disease researchers of any cancer center."[119]

In his second year as an ID fellow, Meyers oversaw a survey study by incoming fellow David Martin of the first 300 transplant patients, looking at whether fungal cultures obtained from urine or sputum or throat swabs were predictive of fungal infections. They were. The two wanted to do a randomized trial on whether a relatively toxic drug could prevent a fungal infection if given prophylactically, but their first findings had been so decisive that it was impossible to do such a trial—the drug was just given prophylactically.

But possibly the most feared infectious complication of bone marrow transplantation was cytomegalovirus, or CMV, a type of herpesvirus. More than half of people in the US harbor CMV, but in people with healthy immune systems, it usually shows no signs or symptoms and does no harm. Meyers's pivotal research showed that CMV was not just present as a bystander in bone marrow transplant deaths, it was the leading infectious killer of transplant patients, responsible for roughly 40 percent of fatalities. In those with suppressed immune systems, the virus can reactivate and cause severe infections and death even months after the transplant.

"When we started, I remember going on rounds and seeing a patient who was otherwise looking fine, listening to their lungs and hearing a few crackles in their lung. It would be CMV," recalled hematologist Fred Appelbaum, who came to work for Thomas in 1978 and went on to become a Fred Hutch deputy director and executive vice president. "And that patient was almost certainly going to die. They went from healthy to dead in a matter of weeks."[120]

Meyers's top priority would be finding an antiviral drug to treat and prevent CMV disease.

David Martin and Lucy Tompkins

King Holmes's training grant—and his growing reputation—led to a boom in fellows. Among them were David H. Martin and Lucy Tompkins, who came to the UW to do residencies. They stayed to do fellowships, starting in 1976, the same year that Walt Stamm returned to the Pacific Northwest. Their careers would take them elsewhere, with the seeds planted during the Seattle years blooming into strong research programs in New Orleans and Palo Alto.

Already intrigued by infectious diseases, Martin had arrived in Seattle to do his residency in 1973, drawn to the UW by Robert Petersdorf's reputation as one of the earliest and best ID specialists in the country. He also was attracted to the collegiality and absence of hierarchy that he saw when he interviewed at the UW.

"People on the West Coast were still very competitive," he said. "But they hid it more than on the East Coast."[121]

He knew that from experience, having graduated from Harvard Medical School and done his internship at Albert Einstein Hospital in New York. He then spent three years at a NIH laboratory in Panama, working primarily on viruses. His mentor there urged him to continue for a PhD, but he chose instead to finish his residency in internal medicine.

In 1975, Martin was one of three people to rotate as chief resident at the Public Health Service Hospital in Seattle, interspersed with heading the emergency and internal medicine departments there. Early on at the UW, Martin figured out that King Holmes was the person to talk to about continuing his training in infectious diseases. The two met, and Holmes seemed supportive of Martin's desire to focus on viruses.

But when he was ready to start his fellowship in 1976, Larry Corey—a year ahead of Martin—had gotten to viruses first. To work with Holmes meant to work on STIs, and Corey was already working on herpes, the only virus then known to be sexually transmitted.

"So King offered me chlamydia, the next best thing—an obligate, intracellular pathogen that couldn't live outside of a cell," Martin said. "It was a bacterium, but pretty close to being like a virus, so maybe I would be happy working with that organism."

In the 1970s, *Chlamydia trachomatis*, like herpes, was considered an emerging pathogen. It was among the smallest bacteria to cause human diseases and vexingly difficult to cultivate in the lab. In a series of studies and papers, Holmes was establishing that it was sexually transmitted.

Early in his fellowship, Martin did the fungal study with Meyers. But over his career, he would become best known for his chlamydia research. At the time, he was just happy that Holmes had offered him a niche and was interested in having him as a fellow—sweetened by the fact that the Public Health Service would continue paying Martin's salary.

Working with Holmes was intense, even if Holmes himself always seemed calm. His intelligence was "overwhelming," Martin said, his enthusiasm infectious. He fostered independence quickly ("Off you go!") but he also encouraged collegiality and being part of a team. His work ethic was phenomenal: During grant-writing season, he would put in 20 hours a day, seven days a week, sleeping on a couch in his office.

Like Holmes, Martin was a Public Health Service officer, and he needed to repay his training by working as a staff physician wherever the PHS needed him. So on New Year's Day 1979, he set out for a job at the PHS hospital in New Orleans.

His departure style befitted his destination: Having stayed up until 4:00 a.m. celebrating New Year's Eve with Seattle friends, he woke up just an hour before his flight. Luckily, there was no airport security in those days to get through.

In New Orleans, he became professor of medicine and of microbiology and chief of infectious diseases at the Louisiana State University School of Medicine. There he ran a chlamydia lab, becoming one of the country's leading experts in that pathogen, and started a Seattle-style STD training and research program.

As fellows moved on across the country and began to develop national and international reputations, it felt, said Martin, like belonging to a club or fraternity. There was not so much competition as pride in each other's accomplishments.

"There was this sense that you wanted to do well and do the best work you could do because you belonged to this group of high-achieving docs who had all trained at the same place," he said. "There was this sense of always wanting to measure up, not only out of camaraderie but of measuring up to the standards that were set by King and others at the UW."

It was Holmes who drew Lucy Tompkins to the UW. While in medical school at Dartmouth, she had come across his work from his Navy years. She was in the library researching *Neisseria* bacteria, which includes gonorrhea. "I started coming across these incredible articles by this guy named King K. Holmes," she said.[122]

The only female in the group of fellows, her path to the UW was far from straightforward.

Tompkins grew up hearing how her mother at age five had survived the 1918 flu epidemic, nursed through her illness by the family doctor. Inspired by that story, Tompkins knew from the time that she was that age that she wanted to be a physician.

But as an undergraduate in biology at Stanford University in the late 1950s, she found little encouragement for women to pursue medical school. She ended up marrying young, transferring to Denver to finish her last year of college, having a child, and then working as a research technician to put her husband through medical school and residency. When he got a job at the NIH, she decided to go to graduate school in immunology at Georgetown University.

There she met Stanley Falkow, then a young professor who had just come over from the NIH and was teaching a course in bacterial genetics. Fascinated by the subject, she switched over to do her doctoral degree with him, despite his misgivings at having a woman— the first—in his lab. Falkow was a gifted mentor, even as he struggled openly with anxiety and agoraphobia early in his career. (It was often said he was more comfortable around microbes than people.) The novelty of having a woman in the lab so flummoxed him that he often didn't even talk to Tompkins.

By the time she had finished her degree three years later, however, her hard work had won his support. When her husband got a job at Dartmouth, it was Falkow who encouraged her to follow her long-postponed dream and enroll in the medical school there. Actually, according to Tompkins, he said: "Stop whining. Just apply, and I'll write you a letter."

She did. When she was accepted, it was so unusual for a 30-year-old woman with an eight-year-old son to be starting medical school that the local newspaper sent out a photographer.

When she learned that Holmes had gone to the University of Washington, that's where she wanted to continue her training. The infectious-diseases field, she said, had long been dominated by (male) researchers on the East Coast—Cornell, the University of Pennsylvania, the University of Virginia, Harvard, Johns Hopkins. The leadership of the Infectious Diseases Society of America predominately came from the East Coast.

Seattle was changing that. Petersdorf already had put the UW on the map for academic medicine. And Kirby's work was well known and respected. "I don't know anyone who didn't love and revere Bill Kirby," Tompkins said.

But what really made the UW known for infectious diseases, she said, was the work of Holmes and his fellows.

"King put Seattle on the global map for sexually transmitted infections. He really resurrected the whole field and made it a big part of infectious diseases," she said. "What put UW on the map was King, Larry, Walt and—in immunocompromised patients—Joel."

It turned out that Tompkins's husband got a job at Seattle's Public Health Service Hospital, and—with another recommendation from Falkow, who was now at the UW—she was able to finish her last year of residency at Harborview. She started an infectious-diseases fellowship in 1976, along with Martin and Stamm, with funding from Holmes's training grant.

Tompkins found her UW years both inspiring and isolating. She was once again older and the sole female in the male-dominated program of that period. Early on, she said, she was told that she had a reputation as being "very hard to work with" because she wasn't interested in research projects suggested by faculty members— including Holmes's suggestion that she investigate whether CMV was sexually transmitted.

But she found a supportive mentor in George Counts, then chief of infectious diseases at Harborview. And she felt welcomed by the other fellows. Corey and Stamm brought her into the monthly gourmet dinner club. She became especially close to Meyers and Thrasher-Meyers. "Joel took me under his wing and invited me to meet Barbara," she said. "I fell in love with both of them. That love sustained me for all these years."

After finishing her infectious-diseases fellowship, Tompkins did a second fellowship in clinical microbiology, working again in Falkow's lab. She and an epidemiologist in the lab, Dennis Schaberg, helped develop a method to identify strains of bacteria in one day rather than weeks. She also began investigating hospital-acquired infections.

Falkow was a generous mentor and a mesmerizing teacher, and a steady stream of infectious-diseases fellows passed through his laboratory and remained friends and colleagues afterward, Corey and Stamm among them. When Falkow left for Stanford in 1981 to head its Department of Microbiology and Immunology, those relationships continued.

Tompkins accepted a position in the UW Department of Laboratory Medicine—albeit with no startup package and an office in the basement, she said. Hers and Falkow's marriages had ended by then, and—after years of avoiding even a hint of a romantic entanglement when she trained with him—they began a relationship after he left the UW. In 1983, she too took a job at Stanford, and they married.

She went on to carve out her own career as chief of Stanford's Division of Infectious Diseases and Geographic Medicine and an associate dean. The post she loved best and has held longest is as chief epidemiologist for Stanford Hospital and Clinics.

"I owe everything to the UW, even though I never would have thrived there as a faculty member," Tompkins said. "You could not find women in leadership positions there. But I treasure the chance that I got to train there. It was a huge, important part of my life."

Under a generation of young, new faculty members—starting with Holmes and continuing with Stamm, Corey, and Meyers—the ID division began to stand out as a welcoming place for women, and women began achieving leadership roles.

Blazing trails

When Walt Stamm returned to the Pacific Northwest in 1976, he had expected to work with Turck on UTIs, which had been Stamm's primary focus at the EIS. He did so, but Turck was spending more time on administrative duties than research, leaving Stamm to look elsewhere for additional mentoring. Holmes stepped in, suggesting that he look for the cause of so-called urethral syndrome, which produced painful and frequent urination in women.

And off Stamm went.

Because it was difficult to get an uncontaminated bacterial sample from women's urine, Stamm developed what David Eschenbach

71

described as an incredible technique for doing a needle punch directly into the bladder. His study found that chlamydia was a significant cause of the syndrome, a finding that bridged Holmes's research on STDs with Turck's in UTIs. Stamm would continue to work in both fields throughout his career—with his trademark calm that made it all seem effortless.

Holmes, Martin, Stamm, and other fellows who followed in chlamydia research worked closely with the leading expert on the bug, Julius Schachter at the University of California, San Francisco. Stamm also credited the UW's Russell Alexander, who studied the neonatal infection of infants by mothers carrying *Chlamydia trachomatis*, with teaching him about "this peculiar organism."[123] In time, among his many influential findings, Stamm would help clarify the role that chlamydia played in causing PID, closing the loop on Eschenbach's and Holmes's earlier influential paper and leading to screening tests that markedly reduced the incidence of PID and the infertility and ectopic pregnancies it can cause.

Stamm finished his fellowship and stayed on as a UW faculty member, continuing to study UTIs and also heading the Chlamydia Research Laboratory at Harborview. Peggy Stamm opened a popular café in their neighborhood of Madison Park. Vivacious and gracious, the couple seemed larger than life, a Seattle version of Jack and Jackie Kennedy in an era that felt like Camelot.

"Walt was amazing in every way," Tompkins said. "He could do anything perfectly, including ski and play tennis."

Corey too, stayed on in Seattle. Near the end of his fellowship, he had a memorable encounter with Robert Petersdorf, who was doing rounds at the Public Health Service Hospital and came across a patient who had endocarditis, his specialty. Noting Corey in the back, Petersdorf said in his throaty growl, "Let me see what the ID fellow said." After reading the young fellow's notes on the patient, he delivered high praise, Petersdorf-style. "Not bad, Corey," he barked.

Soon after, Petersdorf recommended Corey to replace the departing virologist at Seattle Children's Hospital. "This guy's in viral diseases. He's good. Keep him," he told Paul Strandjord, the founding chair of the UW Department of Laboratory Medicine. Strandjord offered Corey a faculty position and became another visionary mentor.

Much as Holmes had done after accepting a job as an epidemiologist in Hawaii, Corey—trained as a physician and at the EIS as an epidemiologist—dashed down to Berkeley to take a course in clinical virology run by California's viral disease laboratory. Six months later, he returned to run the UW virology lab at Seattle Children's. At the time, viruses were mainly seen as problems for children and their treatment the work of pediatricians. To be an internist doing viral research was an anomaly.

But his and Meyers's work was changing that notion. In a few years, HIV would change it even more.

When his fellowship ended, Meyers joined the Fred Hutchinson Cancer Research Center to start a new program that he was inventing as he went. At that time, "there was no field of bone marrow transplantation, let alone infectious diseases in bone marrow transplantation," Corey said.[124]

Barbara Thrasher-Meyers, who loved art and once ran a gallery, set about persuading Northwest photographers to provide landscape prints to hang in the patient-care areas.

"So many patients traveled to Seattle for their treatment and spent their entire stay in hospital rooms, never seeing the beauty of the Northwest," she said. "I thought we could improve patients' spirits by offering them a glimpse of nature."[125]

With Meyers at Fred Hutch, Corey at Seattle Children's, and Stamm at his chlamydia lab at Harborview, the friendships formed in Atlanta grew stronger. The monthly gourmet club dinners rotated among their houses, the wives continued a book club formed in Atlanta, and the Stamm and Corey children played together. Corey and Meyers learned how to ski, following Stamm's tracks—perfect of course—down the Pacific Northwest's towering mountains.

6

STD Research

Booms

Before Sheila A. Lukehart joined King Holmes's growing band of fellows in 1979, she took her first step toward a career in infectious diseases as an undergraduate at the University of California, San Diego. Until then, she had thought her interest in medicine might lead to nursing, the main career path in medicine that seemed open to women when she was growing up. That was before she enrolled in a microbiology class and found out how much fun it was to peer into a microscope.

Sold on research, she headed to graduate studies at UCLA knowing she wanted to focus on bacteria rather than viruses because she wanted to work on something she could see under the microscope. UCLA had just two bacteriologists on the faculty, and the one working on tuberculosis was nearing retirement and no longer taking trainees. So Lukehart checked out the syphilis lab.

"Once I saw syphilis," she said, "I was done making choices."[126]

Partly it was the presence of another woman in the lab, Nancy Bishop, who was finishing up her doctorate as Lukehart was starting out. Bishop became a good friend and an invaluable guide at helping Lukehart get her project set up and navigate graduate school.

But also, the spirochete bacterium, *Treponema pallidum*, just fascinated Lukehart. "I loved watching it under the microscope because it kind of corkscrews around," she said. "It's a difficult bug to work on. You have to grow it in rabbits—you can't cultivate it in a petri dish. So it was a challenge."

It is such a challenge still that today only a handful of laboratories in North America even work on syphilis; Lukehart's among them. Over her career, she became *the* international leader in the biology of *T. pallidum* and the complex relationship between *T. pallidum* and its host.

Syphilis occurs in stages—a primary, a secondary and, after a long period in which it's asymptomatic, a tertiary stage. Before the development of antibiotics, syphilis was a worldwide scourge, largely because of tertiary syphilis.

"There are lots of things that bug has to do in order to evade the immune response," Lukehart said, with just a touch of admiration. "That's where I've focused all of my life: How are these organisms cleared? What happens during secondary syphilis? How does the organism evade the immune system?"

When Lukehart finished her doctorate, her then-husband wanted to move to Seattle to attend a UW graduate program in fisheries. So Lukehart, hearing about Holmes's work, contacted him about an ID fellowship. He had no one working on syphilis and happily welcomed her. Because she needed a place for her rabbits and an animal facility was still under construction, she first did a year-long fellowship at UC San Diego, where she studied rabbit immunology, before arriving in Seattle in July 1979.

Holmes, she said, "pushed people to try new things, to go in different directions." What she remembers of her first meeting with him was that he advised her from the get-go to write a grant. When she said she couldn't write a grant because she wasn't on faculty, he told her that winning a grant would get her an appointment. So she wrote—and won—a grant with Holmes as a co-investigator. And she got her faculty appointment.

Two other women had been on the ID faculty when Lukehart started her fellowship, but both left soon after—Elaine Jong to head the UW student health services and Joan Knapp to the CDC's gonorrhea laboratory.

After Jong and Knapp left, Lukehart was the only woman at faculty meetings. Also, most of the ID faculty had medical degrees and were on a different career track from research faculty with PhDs like her. "It wasn't very comfortable," she said. "But I guess I'm not one to mince words. I say what I think. And I spoke up when I thought I needed to speak up."

At the Public Health Hospital, however, where the STD research—and many of the younger faculty and fellows were concentrated—Lukehart felt at home. And Knapp—who was also a PhD—was still there working with Holmes on gonorrhea and kept a playpen in her lab for her young children. New classes of fellows that followed included more women, many of whom stayed on and joined the faculty.

Holmes was Lukehart's primary mentor. Like everyone else, she remembers as a fellow waiting—sometimes for hours—beyond a scheduled appointment time to meet with him but having his undivided attention during the meeting. And like every other fellow, she spent countless afternoons going over every sentence in manuscripts with him, heeding his suggestions to tweak the paper's tone by dropping a word here or changing a word there.

"He's a great writer," she said. "And he spent the time with his trainees, early on, to make us good writers too."

She also said that he was always adamant about giving credit to his trainees. She did laboratory rather than clinical work, and her first manuscript was a basic science paper. She put Holmes's name on it because, besides being her mentor, he had supported the research financially. "This is your work," he told her, striking his name off. "You have to fly on your own."

"He was a fabulous mentor," she said. "He continues to be. He counts you as his kids forever."

The "kids" in training with Lukehart included a raft of outstanding fellows who did not stay at the UW but became leading researchers in their own areas and took the "Seattle method" around the country and the world. They included Edward W. "Ned" Hook III, who was the son of Robert Petersdorf's good friend from his training days at Johns Hopkins; Canadian Robert Brunham; Belgian Peter Piot; and Thomas Quinn.

All of them—Lukehart, Hook, Brunham, Piot, and Quinn—would go on to receive the American STD Association's Distinguished Career Award, following in the footsteps of Larry Corey, Walt Stamm, and Holmes himself.

As would an earlier fellow—Hunter Handsfield—who returned to the UW during this period.

The "Seattle model"

After delaying the doctor draft until he had finished his ID fellowship, Hunter Handsfield entered the Navy and was stationed in San Diego. He returned to Seattle in 1978 to head the Sexually Transmitted Disease Control Program for the Seattle–King County Public Health Department. Shortly after taking the position, he closed the old venereal diseases, or VD, clinic—an increasingly out-of-date term used before the 1970s that implied venery, or immoral behavior—and moved all the services over to Harborview Medical Center. He took over from King Holmes as director of the STD clinic there, becoming the first director to be jointly appointed by the university and the county.

The "Seattle model" of bridging public health services and academic research was underway.

The Seattle–King County STD Control Program became one of the first public health programs in the nation to expand prevention efforts beyond syphilis and gonorrhea to include emerging syndromes such as genital herpes, chlamydial infections, and other STIs. Handsfield also established a practice, revolutionary at the time, of using physician assistants and nurse practitioners to provide comprehensive clinical and prevention services.

At the same time, he continued his academic research, focusing primarily on asymptomatic gonococcal infections and the emergence and epidemiology of resistant gonococcal infections to antibiotics. He led single and multicenter clinical trials for the treatment of gonorrhea, syphilis, and chlamydia. New fellows moved through the clinic, working on their own research projects. It was a no-silos world; Walt Stamm's laboratory handled specimens from the lab.

"We proved that, when properly done, academic research enhances clinical care rather than interferes with it and that people in academics can develop mutually beneficial, collegial relationships with people in public health institutions," Handsfield said.[127]

Many years later, Ned Hook described the impact of Handsfield's work when he introduced Handsfield as the 2010 recipient of the American Sexually Transmitted Diseases Association's Distinguished Career Award (formerly Thomas Parran Award).[128]

"The STD control program at Seattle–King County Health Department in combination with the University of Washington has served as the model for health departments across the United States," said Hook, a UW resident and fellow in the 1970s. "Many of us who trained with Dr. Handsfield tried to employ variations of this model and many others aspired to do so. Fundamental to this model was the idea that the association of public health and academic research was a win-win: both sides could benefit, and patients benefitted."[129]

The role of Harborview

The establishment of the STD clinic at Harborview—and the closing, a decade later, of the US Public Health Service Hospital—marked the ascendancy of Harborview Medical Center as a hub of ID research, primarily the STD work undertaken by Holmes and his growing cadre of fellows.

Holmes himself was still based at the Public Health Service Hospital, where he and his fellows had pretty much taken over the 11th floor. But the federal government had been making noises about closing PHS hospitals since the Eisenhower administration, and in 1981, President Reagan sounded the death knell. Local efforts to save the hospital under city management—it was renamed Pacific Medical Center, or PacMed—kept it open for another few years. Holmes, his fellows, their laboratories, and their clinics all moved to Harborview by 1984, the year Holmes became chief of medicine there.

To Handsfield, basing STD research at Harborview contributed to Seattle's growing expertise as a center of STD—and later HIV/AIDS—studies. The UW-operated county medical center was located closer to the populations hardest hit by STDs and later by HIV/AIDS, contributing to a sense of urgency and pushing the researchers to work all the harder.

Harborview had been a key clinical training site since the founding of the UW School of Medicine. In the beginning, the county owned and ran Harborview as King County Hospital, with students and residents rotating through. In 1967, the university and King County entered into an agreement for the UW to take over clinical management of the hospital, with all physicians recognized as academic faculty. Still, Harborview retained its mission as a county hospital for underserved populations.

While such collaborations between universities and county or city hospitals are common nationwide, in Seattle, the association between the two institutions was and remains unique. Although still owned by King County, hospital operations are solely the responsibility of the university, which employs all personnel, both professional and supportive. The working agreement with the county required the university to provide care regardless of patients' financial resources or social station.

The division of labor could be roughly summed up as pregnant women at UW Medical Center, gunshot victims at Harborview. The STD clinic, naturally, wound up at Harborview. In fact, the STD population was named as a priority group in the county's working agreement.

Marvin Turck helped shape the Harborview culture as chief of infectious diseases there in the 1960s and chief of medicine in the 1970s.

"Those people who came to Harborview came there because they enjoyed taking care of the under-served," Turck said. "The Harborview mission is still quite different from the University of Washington's."[130]

Harborview maintained a distinct institutional personality, including a reputation as a place where the house staff had a great degree of autonomy and responsibility. ("Off you go!") Ned Hook arrived in Seattle in 1976 to start his residency at Harborview, where Turck was chief of medicine. He later served as Turck's chief resident.

"Harborview is where the action was—the busiest ICU, the sickest patients, the ward service where house officers had the most independence," Hook said. "That, combined with the group of people who were at Harborview, provided an extraordinary opportunity."[131]

Chief among that group was Turck, whose love of and skill at teaching were evident. "His presence, his confidence, his font of knowledge were inspiring to us," Hook said.

Turck's devotion to Harborview extended to helping run bond campaigns to raise the community funding needed to operate the medical center. "I was very good at passing bond issues for Harborview," he said. "I was a good politician."[132]

Edward W. Hook III

Back when he started medical school at Cornell University, Ned Hook had not intended to follow in the footsteps of his father, who had trained with Petersdorf at Johns Hopkins and was a founding member and president of the Infectious Diseases Society of America. It was Merle Sande, a mentee and friend of his father's and also a legendary infectious-diseases physician-researcher, who sold the younger Hook on the field.

Known for his personal charm and his enthusiasm for his work, Sande invited Ned Hook to go duck hunting over the Christmas holidays. Sande then asked the medical school freshman about his summer plans and casually offered a job in his lab. Hook accepted and found the research on bacterial endocarditis so intriguing he returned for the next two summers, publishing papers in the process.

Sande had earned his medical degree at the University of Washington—he had grown up in Washington state, where his father was a Puget Sound ferry boat captain—and recommended that Hook apply to do his residency there. Sande himself returned to Seattle in 2005 as an ID professor after a storied career that included being chair of medicine at San Francisco General Hospital and founding the first hospital ward in the world for the diagnosis and treatment of AIDS; establishing a research program and an infectious-diseases institute at Makerere University in Kampala, Uganda; and serving as chair of medicine at the University of Utah School of Medicine.

When Ned Hook arrived in Seattle in 1976 to do his internal medicine residency, his father, by then chair of medicine at the University of Virginia, was involved in a public—if friendly—disagreement with his old friend Petersdorf over whether infectious-diseases specialists had a role outside of academic research. Petersdorf argued that there was no need for ID specialists in private practice; in just a few years, he would go further and publish his article arguing that too many specialists were being trained, period, and singling out infectious diseases as an example.

But Hook was undeterred. While serving as Turck's chief resident in 1979–1980, he started looking into doing an ID fellowship. Wanting laboratory experience, he began working on gonorrhea, chlamydia, and syphilis with Handsfield, Stamm, and Lukehart.

"Seattle was the center of the STD world at that time," Hook said. "It was inhabited by young people who were approachable, easy to communicate with, highly productive and highly interactive. King had recruited people who would have a large impact on the program. A lot of new knowledge was being generated."[133]

What impressed Hook was not just the caliber of people that Holmes attracted but how they worked together. Meetings on the 11th floor of the Public Health Hospital would draw Larry Corey, Walt Stamm, and Hunter Handsfield alongside the infectious-diseases fellows. Because STD syndromes—PID, vaginal discharge, urethral discharge, proctitis—could be caused by so many different pathogens, Holmes tapped Handsfield's clinical expertise, Stamm's knowledge of chlamydia, and Corey for herpesvirus.

"You've got a bunch of big personalities with a lot on the ball and a lot to bring to the table—and they all pitch in," Hook said. "Seattle had the appropriate critical mass to conduct such research, and one of King's many gifts was to be able to promote effective, highly productive collaborations to provide comprehensive answers."[134]

More than big-name physician-researchers had a seat at the table. Before Seattle, Hook would do a study and then call in a statistician to work up the results. Holmes flipped that typical pattern by bringing statisticians in early to help determine what a study needed to show and how many participants were needed to show it. He set up teams that included nurse practitioners, laboratorians, epidemiologists, and statisticians.

Everyone who played a crucial role on the study was listed as an author on published papers, the power currency of academic medicine. That was different too. The norm when Hook was in medical school was two or three authors at most.

It was not just a matter of Holmes acknowledging every team member's research contributions and giving credit where credit was due, though it was that as well. The comprehensive, all-hands-on-deck approach translated to better treatments for patients.

"King really promoted the area of team science," Hook said. "Many of us who followed have done our best to emulate this highly effective team approach to our research, but it was not common before King led the way."[135]

Robert Brunham

When Robert C. Brunham arrived in Seattle in 1978 to spend three years as an infectious-diseases fellow, he sought out King Holmes intentionally to study STDs. The days of fellows coming close to fainting at hearing the subject of Holmes's research were (almost) over.

A native of Creston, British Columbia, Brunham earned his medical degree from the University of British Columbia and trained in internal medicine and microbiology at McGill University in Montreal. During training, he had been called down to the emergency room to see a young woman suffering from acute PID. She had lower abdominal pain and symptoms of gonorrhea, which was confirmed in the lab. Her male partner had no symptoms but also tested positive.

"I was so struck by that—not only the medical problem but the epidemiological link, the transmission link, the public health link," Brunham said. "I began to read about that topic and came across King's publications."[136]

Holmes was developing a national reputation by then. He had just gotten a major NIH grant. And far from sending someone out to see who this young upstart was, as had happened when he applied for his first training grant, his NIH reviewers declared him a national treasure.

He was certainly that to Brunham, who arrived at age 30 with his wife and newborn son, feeling a little out of his depth as a fledgling researcher. Holmes helped him get settled, even giving him his used car.

"He was larger than life to me," Brunham said. "Physically, he is not a large person. But when you're in his company, you can feel the gravity of him as a person. The two cardinal characteristics of King are the sheer power of his rational intellect and his amazing social intelligence."

Holmes was not the only larger-than-life person Brunham encountered in Seattle. He attended lectures by microbiologist Stan Falkow and rotated through the bone marrow transplantation center run by Don Thomas. And to work under Petersdorf and Beeson was to be in the presences of "the founding fathers of infectious diseases," Brunham said. He described Petersdorf as "opinionated and declarative." Beeson "had a touch of royalty in him when he spoke and gave rounds."

Brunham particularly remembered a talk Beeson gave on physicians who had won the Nobel Prize. "He told that story as the great arc of medical history," he said. "His knowledge of the medical literature was encyclopedic." (Lukehart agreed, recalling a lecture on Beeson's father's 1925 dogsled run to Nome with diphtheria antitoxin.)

However, Brunham strongly disagreed with Petersdorf on one subject. He arrived the year that Petersdorf had shocked his fellow infectious-diseases researchers by publishing the article opining that too many ID specialists were being trained.

"He was looking at ID in the pre-Holmes way, having to do with people who came into the hospital with life-threatening infections," Brunham said. "King had this more ecological, holistic concept of infections and an interest in sexually transmitted infections. Now of course we see infectious diseases in line with public health and have moved beyond simply their treatment to their prevention and control. King really took the field in a different, broader direction."

And then there was Turck, who remained renowned for his teaching—and for his recognition of and support for others' talents, including Holmes's prodigious research skills.

"That's what King brought that was different from Marvin," Brunham said. "I could take any of my research data to King, who would of course know less about the data than I did. But he would look at it and interpret it in ways I never could. He would connect the dots, see the patterns. That's what made Marvin appreciate King so much. Marvin created the opportunities for King to take root in Seattle."

In Seattle, working with and learning from Walt Stamm and David Martin, Brunham began the research that would make him an internationally recognized expert in chlamydia. He focused on acquiring skills in chlamydia biology and pathogenesis in the laboratory of microbiologist San-pin Wang. Born in Taiwan, San-pin had emigrated to Seattle in 1964 to work with epidemiologist J. Thomas Grayston, who later became the founding dean of the UW School of Public Health. The two began collaborating in 1958, when Grayston was head of the Department of Microbiology at the US Naval Medical Research Unit-2 in Taipei. In 1970, San-pin developed the micro-immunofluorescence test, the first type-specific serologic test for laboratory diagnosis of chlamydial infection.[137] Using the test, he and his colleagues—including Holmes, Handsfield, Turck, and

Russ Alexander—were able in 1975 to define chlamydia as a sexually transmitted pathogen.[138]

But looming over them all, both professionally and personally, was Holmes.

"He is extraordinary in the way he can connect with people immediately and make relationships that allow you to have discussions about medicine, about books you have read, about current events," Brunham said. "He lives his life in a very full and completely positive manner—he almost never talks badly about anything or anyone."

Peter Piot

Holmes was also the draw for Peter Piot, who arrived in Seattle to train with him the same year as Brunham. Piot in 1978 already had a considerable accomplishment to his name: two years earlier, when he was just 27 years old, he had codiscovered the Ebola virus.

Growing up in a small town in Belgium, Piot's interest in infectious diseases, stigma, and social justice was first sparked by the local hero, Father Damien, a Flemish missionary who ministered to a colony of lepers in Molokai, Hawaii.

Like Brunham, Piot was undeterred by professors who said that antibiotics had conquered infectious diseases. (Petersdorf was far from alone in this view.) He combined medical school at the University of Ghent with a diploma in tropical medicine at the Institute of Tropical Medicine in Antwerp. While in Antwerp, he worked in a clinic for travelers and sailors, which ended up being the de facto STD clinic, while continuing graduate studies in microbiology.

He also trained as a pathologist, and in 1976, he tested a sample of blood from a missionary nun who had died in Zaire (now the Democratic Republic of Congo). Everyone suspected that she had died from yellow fever, but the virus that the Antwerp team, of which Piot was a junior member, isolated was definitely not that. Specimens were also sent to the CDC, which confirmed that it was a new virus. Soon Piot found himself on a plane to Zaire with researchers from the CDC and elsewhere to investigate whether the virus was connected to a deadly epidemic of hemorrhagic fever occurring there. It was, and subsequently the disease and the virus were named for the Ebola River flowing near the epidemic's epicenter.

Piot had become interested in STIs both in Antwerp and while working on Ebola in Zaire, where he saw an epidemic of STDs as well as many women with infertility related to PID. Looking through the medical literature, he found Holmes.

"King Holmes was the first one to take a systematic, scientifically rigorous approach to the study of STDs," Piot said. "It is definitely through his leadership that sexually transmitted infections have gained scientific respectability."[139]

After Zaire, the CDC invited Piot to Atlanta, and he found a NATO fellowship to pay for his travel. There, he finished the six-week EIS boot camp but found the CDC too bureaucratic. So he bought a car and drove across the country to Seattle with his wife and young son in tow, hoping to convince Holmes to take him on as a fellow.

Everyone has a story of their first meeting with Holmes. Piot, invited for lunch, arrived at his soon-to-be-mentor's home to find Holmes in the kitchen making peanut butter sandwiches. A man on the roof was trying to get the TV antenna in the right position; Piot's job was to stand outside the house, relaying directions from Holmes to the TV repair person.

Apparently, he passed inspection. (Ebola aside, it helped that he brought his own funding.) Piot ended up working with Holmes on bacterial vaginosis, which didn't yet have a name. Holmes also introduced him to Stanley Falkow, and Piot learned to work on plasmids in Falkow's laboratory, sharing a bench with Lucy Tompkins. It was a time of "total revolution" [140] in microbiology, Piot said. PCR did not yet exist, but researchers at the UW were preparing western blots and other new techniques. Genetic sequencing was just starting.

Piot, like Hook, was especially impressed by the way Holmes built multidisciplinary groups of microbiologists, statisticians, clinicians, epidemiologists, and social scientists to work a problem from all angles—a model Piot would follow throughout his career.

"It was a life-changing experience for me, not so much in terms of knowledge but in *how* to work," he said. "The sky seemed to be the limit."[141]

Piot learned from young faculty members as well, such as Larry Corey, who was doing original work on herpes.

"Again, for me, it was a whole new world that opened," Piot said. "Larry had very solid lab science underpinning what he was doing, but also they went into super detail in terms of people's sex lives. The approach was really an eye-opener for me—the commitment to find the solution to the issues and also making sure you used the best science to find the solution."

Plus, he added, "We laughed a lot also, which I think is important."[142]

Bob Brunham, whose fellowship overlapped with Piot's and who became a good friend, introduced Piot to Allan Ronald. After training at the UW a decade earlier under Marvin Turck and John Sherris, Ronald had returned to his native Canada to direct the clinical microbiology program at the University of Manitoba. His dean and chair of medicine initially saw little need for his infectious-diseases training, so convinced were they that sanitation, vaccines, and antibiotics had made the subfield unnecessary. Ronald persevered, continuing the research into the pathogenesis and management of UTIs that he had begun under Turck and building Manitoba into a center of expertise in that area.

In the mid-1970s, he further proved the value of his ID training when Winnipeg clinics began seeing an unusually high number of patients with painful genital ulcers. Ronald and one of his fellows, Greg Hammond, identified the outbreak as a STD known as chancroid. They traced the outbreak to sex workers, and once they got the women into treatment, were able to end the epidemic and eradicate chancroid from Winnipeg.

Brunham, knowing that Piot had experience isolating the bacterium involved, connected the two men, and Ronald invited Piot to Winnipeg to give a talk. Ronald himself had just returned from Nairobi. A paper he published on the Winnipeg outbreak had caught the attention of Herbert Nsanze, a microbiologist heading the University of Nairobi's Department of Medical Microbiology, who contacted Ronald about problems with chancroid and other STDs in Kenya. At the invitation of Nsanze and the World Health Organization (WHO), Ronald visited Nairobi. It was the beginning of what would become a decades-long research collaboration, with Holmes and other UW researchers, along with former fellows such as Brunham and Piot, deeply involved.

"It was kind of a domino effect, or a chain reaction, from one connection to the other," Piot said of his year at the UW.[143]

Over the next three decades, Piot would also work frequently with Corey and with a new fellow, Tom Quinn, who arrived at the

UW in 1979, as they all became immersed in the epidemic of their lifetimes, HIV/AIDS.

Thomas Quinn

Tom Quinn looked at several infectious-diseases fellowship programs before choosing the UW because King Holmes convinced him it was one of the best programs and he would do well in it. It was and he did, even if it wasn't what he'd initially expected.

With a master's degree in parasitology from the University of Notre Dame, a medical degree from Northwestern University, and training in internal medicine at Albany Medical Center in New York, Quinn had spent the past two years at the NIH's Laboratory of Parasitic Diseases. He came to the UW in 1979 thinking he would continue to pursue his research interest in malaria.

When he told Holmes that during their first conversation, his new mentor replied, "Well, malaria's not sexually transmitted."

Quinn was just about to explain how malaria had a sexual cycle—or the parasite did, anyway—when Holmes's phone rang. He was on call that night, and the resident on duty—who happened to be Ned Hook—wanted help with a patient who had "rip-roaring proctitis."

Knowing that many gay patients who had been seen in the STD clinic were infected with parasites, Holmes told Quinn, "I want you to go work this guy up."

So off Quinn went.

"On day one, I was thrown immediately into it," Quinn said. "We worked him up. The specimens went to Walt [Stamm's] lab. Within two weeks of my arrival, I was fully active in my research project."[144]

That particular patient turned out to be infected not with parasites but with chlamydia, but, like erstwhile virologist David Martin before him, Quinn took some comfort in the wily bacterium's resemblance to the pathogen he had previously studied. At the two-week marker, Holmes called a meeting of young faculty members Quinn called "giants in the field, or they were becoming giants"—Stamm, Larry Corey, Hunter Handsfield, Russ Alexander, and dermatologist Jim Harnisch. An hour of feedback and advice followed.

"That meeting I will never forget—it was the way it worked in

Seattle," Quinn said. "How was I going to do this project? I had to go into the clinic and work under Hunter. I was to collect samples of chlamydia—that's Walt's lab. I was to do herpes. That was Larry's. To be successful, you couldn't be in a silo. I was off and running with a big project on infections in men who have sex with men."

In the clinic, Handsfield took Quinn under his wing, mentoring him in clinical examination skills. Seeing how productive Quinn's project was turning out to be, Handsfield assigned him a physician assistant, Manny Mkrtichian, to continue the clinical work, and Quinn moved back into the laboratory and started writing papers. "Having that kind of support mechanism for a fellow—that was remarkable," Quinn said.

He found himself as intrigued by the infections he was studying as he had been with malaria. He did find a wide range of parasitic infections, sped along by a gay liberation movement that led to certain sex practices becoming more common, such as oral-rectal sex and "fisting," or inserting a fist into the partner's rectum and causing rectal or colonic injuries. Such practices may have been new to him as a straight man (and yet another Notre Dame graduate), but Quinn's focus was on the new syndromes he was finding. "I was into the discovery and the science," he said.

By the late 1970s, STD clinics in Seattle and elsewhere began seeing an assortment of chronic infections of the anus and lower gut they called gay bowel syndrome. Quinn, Stamm, Corey, and Holmes published a key early paper on these intestinal infections in the *New England Journal of Medicine*.

Other infectious-diseases divisions were not yet tied into county STD clinics the way the UW was.

"We have King and Hunter to thank for making that work," Quinn said. "You couldn't do the kind of research I was asked to do unless you were linked to these clinics. A lot of the divisions today modeled their association with STD clinics after the Seattle model. Seattle is where it all took off."

The sense of collaboration and collegiality extended throughout the division. Seymour Klebanoff was the head of the ID division during Quinn's fellowship years. Knowing that Quinn had spent the past two years working in an NIH basic science laboratory, Klebanoff opened his lab to him, saying, "If you're interested at some point, you'd be welcome to come to my lab, come to my seminars, see what we're doing."

"Seymour was one of those people you could sit with and talk about science or world events, it didn't really matter," Quinn said. "He was cordial, friendly, warm, just a person you could easily talk to."

Others were equally welcoming. At a picnic for newcomers, Quinn met pediatrician and immunologist Chris Wilson, who had just joined the UW faculty, and became intrigued by Wilson's research on macrophages. And Quinn shared a laboratory with Sheila Lukehart, who began her fellowship under Holmes the same year Quinn did and taught him how to work with rabbits.

"She's the leading person in syphilis research today. Having shared a lab with her was really exciting," Quinn said. "The work environment—who you shared a lab with—really mattered."

At that point, six or more fellows were coming in each year, for a total of 12 over the two years of an average fellowship.

"It's not always the faculty, it's also the peers. The people you're working with can have a major influence on how you do work and how you move forward," Quinn said. "Because we were compatriots, we would get together and talk and share ideas. And that's what makes for fertile ground."

Because Quinn shared a lab with Lukehart just down the hall from Holmes's office, he developed a strategy for dealing with how far behind Holmes ran on appointments. Quinn would ask for a 6:00 p.m. time slot, then just keep an eye on Holmes's door. His mentor rarely went home before 8:00 p.m. or 9:00 p.m., so Quinn could usually squeeze in.

Quinn had his share of Holmes rewrites.

"Remember, it was all done on a typewriter," he said. "He didn't just redo it and send it back to you in track changes. And he always wrote in a scrawl—it was very difficult to read his handwriting. But since you're there listening to him, he would explain what he was doing. You would watch him take sentence by sentence and rewrite it. Although we laugh about it now, it was very important that we learned that process."

Quinn's training was not entirely focused on STDs. Both he and Holmes were in the Public Health Service at that time and would occasionally be called up on an emergency basis. The Cuban "boat people" refugee crisis peaked during Quinn's fellowship years. Refugees fleeing Vietnam after the war's end were sent to Fort Chaffee, Arkansas—where Elvis had undergone basic training, Quinn noted—and Holmes was called up to staff the medical service.

The call came at the height of a very hot, very humid Arkansas summer. When Holmes found out just one officer was needed, he suggested that another PHS officer—a fellow under him—go in his place. Quinn rolled with it.

He also did a stint with bone marrow transplant patients, learning to treat infections in severely immunocompromised patients. "Where else could an ID fellow get that experience in 1979?" he said. "Nowhere but here. It was brand-new then. Now it's all over the place."

An award and departures

While King Holmes was training dozens of fellows and establishing STD research as an academic field, Bill Kirby and others remained actively involved in infectious-diseases research and teaching at the UW Medical Center. In 1977, Kirby received the Bristol Award from the Infectious Diseases Society of America, the most prestigious award in the field.

In 1979, Robert Petersdorf left his position as chair of UW Medicine to serve as president of a Brigham and Women's Hospital in Boston, a new Harvard teaching facility that combined four area hospitals. In 1981, he became vice chancellor for health sciences and dean of the School of Medicine at UC San Diego, where he served for five years. From 1986 to 1994, Petersdorf headed the Association of American Medical Colleges (AAMC).

"I learned from him academic citizenship," said Marvin Turck of his mentor. "He was very driving. Being chairman of medicine was not sufficient for him, so he subsequently became the dean at San Diego and was president of the AAMC. He's a legendary person in infectious diseases."[145]

It would not be the last Seattle would see of Petersdorf.

Two earlier ID fellows, David Martin and Lucy Tompkins, left Seattle around the same period, he to Louisiana State University School of Medicine in 1979 and she to Stanford in 1983.

Sheila Lukehart stayed on, not only becoming internationally recognized for her studies of syphilis but eventually taking over from Holmes directing the UW STD & HIV Research Training Program and serving as an associate dean for research and graduate education.

But many of the cohorts she trained with during those busy years in the late 1970s and early 1980s moved on.

After his fellowship, Robert Brunham moved to Winnipeg, recruited—at Holmes's recommendation—by fellow Canadian Allan Ronald. Holmes often said he should never have let the Brunhams escape Seattle.[146] But, as with most of his departing fellows, their collaboration would continue.

Peter Piot returned to Antwerp, where in 1981 he, like infectious-diseases researchers around the world, read a CDC report about five gay men suffering from an unknown syndrome that was wiping out their immune system. Like so many of King's fellows, he dedicated the next decades of his career to HIV/AIDS.

When he finished his two-year fellowship, Tom Quinn, like Martin, went where the Public Health Service needed him to repay their support for his training. The PHS sent him to Baltimore. Shortly afterward, he recruited Ned Hook there to set up the "Seattle model" of cooperation between academic researchers and county STD clinics. Hook then took the Seattle method to Birmingham when he moved there to head infectious diseases at the University of Alabama.

In a few years, Quinn too would become a key player in the nation's response to the AIDS epidemic—a role he attributes to the serendipity of that first assignment on his first day meeting with Holmes, the mentor he later dubbed "the king of sexually transmitted infections."

"Looking at this epidemic of STIs in gay men was not what I had trained in—I was a malaria immunologist," he said. "But at the end of the two-year fellowship, boom, the AIDS epidemic occurs, it's only being described in men who have sex with men, it's a sexually transmitted infection—and that was exactly what I'd worked on."[147]

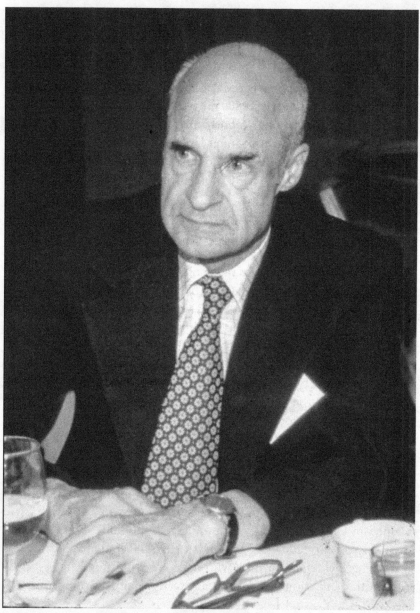

William Kirby arrived in Seattle in 1949 as the first infectious-diseases specialist in the Pacific Northwest. One of the original members of the UW Department of Medicine, he was an expert in tuberculosis and other chest diseases and a leader of the antibiotic revolution. *Photo courtesy of the University of Washington*

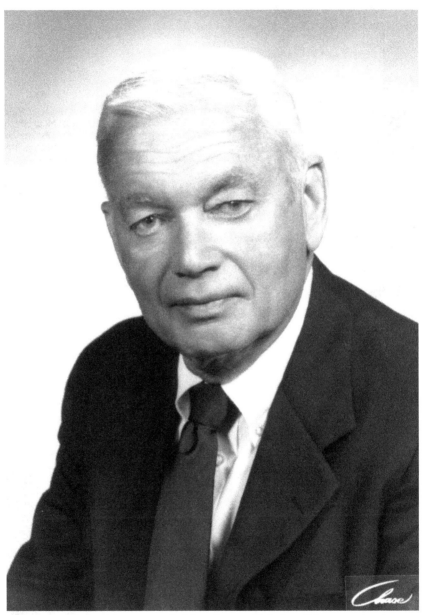

Robert Petersdorf was known as a builder. First as chief of medicine at Harborview and then as UW chair of medicine from 1964–1979, he attracted stellar faculty and fellows. *Photo copyright © 2006 AAMC*

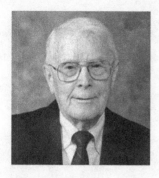

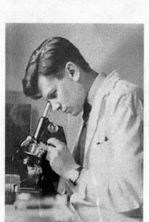

(Top) Paul Beeson was Petersdorf's mentor at Yale and later a VA Distinguished Professor of Medicine in Seattle. A pioneering infectious diseases researcher, he was equally renowned for his patient care. *Jay Gross Photography/AFAR, 2006*

(Middle) John Sherris, an expert in what was then called clinical bacteriology, came from England in 1959 to run the microbiology laboratory program at the newly opened UW School of Medicine. *Photo courtesy of the University of Washington*

(Bottom) Seymour Klebanoff, one of the best white-blood cell researchers in the world, revolutionized science's understanding of the body's infection-fighting immune system. He led the ID division from 1976–1994. *Photo courtesy of the University of Washington*

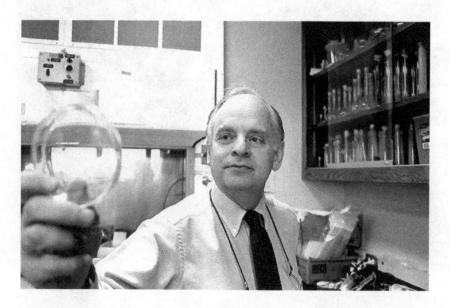

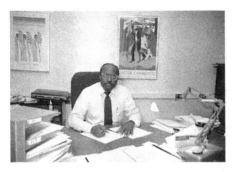

(Above) George Counts, recruited as a fellow by Marvin Turck in 1965, became ID chief at Harborview, then director of the clinical microbiology lab at Fred Hutch. He was known throughout the country as an extraordinary mentor for minority physician-researchers. *Photo by Richard Wilhelm, Fred Hutchinson Cancer Research Center*

(Right) When King Holmes arrived in Seattle in 1967 to do his residency, he had already begun his transformative research into sexually transmitted infections as epidemiologist for the US 7th Fleet in the Western Pacific. *Photo courtesy of King Holmes*

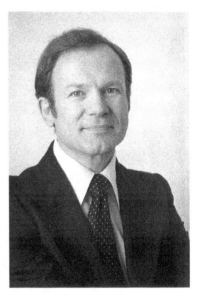

(Bottom left) Marvin Turck first came to Seattle in 1960 as an officer in the Epidemic Intelligence Service and trained as a fellow with Petersdorf. His research focused primarily on urinary tract infections, but what he loved most was the clinical practice and teaching of medicine. *Photo by H. Hunter Handsfield*

(Bottom right) The Kirby-Bauer-Sherris-Turck single-disk diffusion method, developed in the late 1950s and early 1960s to determine a pathogen's susceptibility or resistance before prescribing an antibiotic, is still in use. *Photo courtesy of the University of Washington*

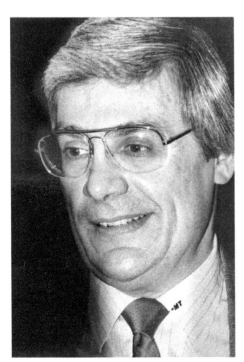

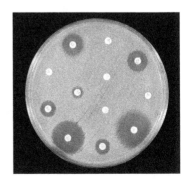

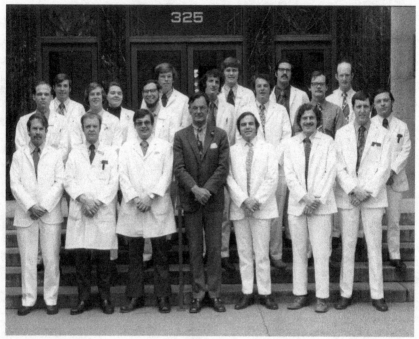

Walt Stamm (fourth row, left) first met mentor Marvin Turck (front row, third from left) while a UW resident in internal medicine in the early 1970s. *Photo courtesy of the University of Washington*

King Holmes (second from left) mentored more than 150 fellows during a career spanning five decades. Among them was David Martin (far right), who was as an ID fellow from 1976–1979, focusing on chlamydia. *Photo by H. Hunter Handsfield*

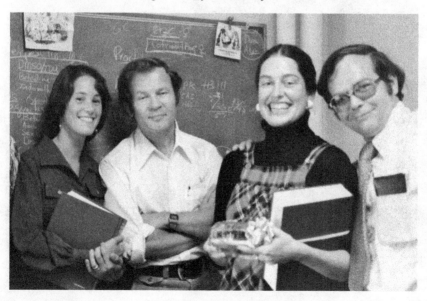

After training as an ID fellow with King Holmes from 1975–1977, Larry Corey opened a lab at Seattle Children's Hospital. He sealed his reputation as a force in infectious diseases early on by leading clinical trials on the world's first antiviral therapy, acyclovir, to control and suppress genital herpes. These early studies paved the way for antiviral therapies for HIV, as well as for hepatitis B and C. Later, Corey turned to the biggest challenge of all—working to develop a preventive vaccine against HIV. *Photo courtesy of Larry Corey*

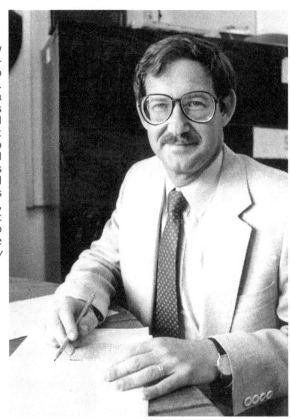

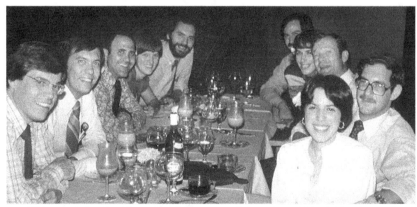

In addition to their scientific accomplishments, ID fellows forged friendships that endured. King Holmes (right, center) titled this snapshot "The young lions." To his left are Larry Corey and Carol Spiegel, and across the table are (from front to back) Walt Stamm, Hunter Handsfield, Ken Wagner, Pat Totten, and Peter Piot. *Photo courtesy of King Holmes*

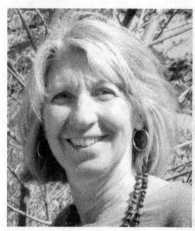

Sheila Lukehart joined King Holmes' growing band of fellows in 1979. She already had begun the research that would make her one of the world's experts on syphilis. *Photo courtesy of University of Washington*

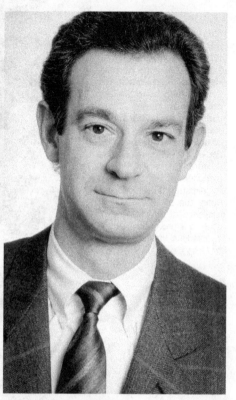

(Right) Joel Meyers spent the 1980s launching the first program in the country to study and treat the unique infections that plague bone marrow transplant patients. In 1991, he died of colon cancer at age 46, weeks before his landmark paper on ganciclovir and CMV was published. *Photo courtesy of Fred Hutchinson Cancer Research Center*

(Below, and right) An ID fellow in 1976, Lucy Tompkins was one of the first women in the program. Joel Meyers, who began his ID fellowship a year earlier, became a close and supportive friend. She went on to become chief of Stanford's Division of Infectious Diseases and Geographic Medicine and chief epidemiologist for Stanford Hospital and Clinics. *Photos courtesy of Lucy Tompkins*

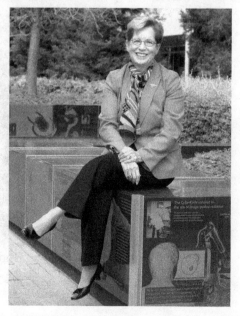

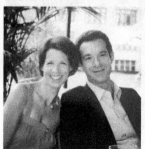

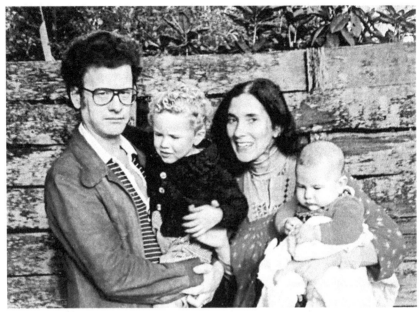

Canadian Robert Brunham studied chlamydia as a fellow under King Holmes, arriving with his young family in 1978. Holmes, he recalled, was "larger than life" and helped him get settled, even giving him a used car. *Photo courtesy of King Holmes*

Seattle-trained ID researchers who focused on chlamydia gathered for a conference at Sweden's Örenäs Castle in 1982. From left to right: Swedish researcher Per-Anders Mårdh; David Eschenbach; King Holmes (in hat); Peter Piot; Walt Stamm; Tom Quinn; Pat Totten; and Mike Lovett, a UW fellow who went on to UCLA. *Photo courtesy of King Holmes*

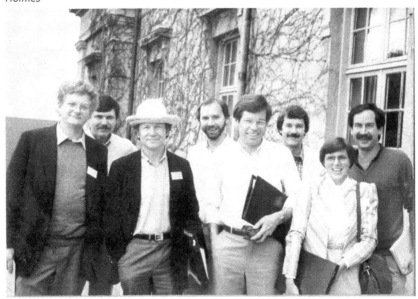

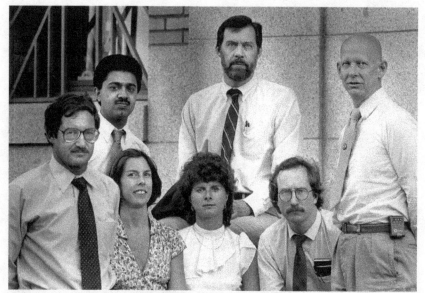

Seattle researchers in 1986 won one of the first NIH grants to test AIDS drugs and treatment. Pictured clockwise from left: team leader Larry Corey; UW pharmaceutics researcher Jash Unadkat; Hunter Handsfield; Bob Wood; Bob Coombs; UW pharmaceutics researcher Teresa Tartaglione; and Ann Collier. *Photo by Alan Berner, staff photographer,* The Seattle Times

Ned Hook, left, and Walt Stamm both served as chief residents under Marvin Turck and trained as ID fellows with King Holmes. Hook went on to direct the Division of Infectious Diseases at the University of Alabama, Birmingham. Stamm led the ID division at the UW from 1994–2007. *Photo courtesy of King Holmes*

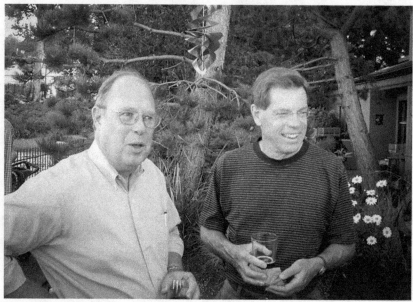

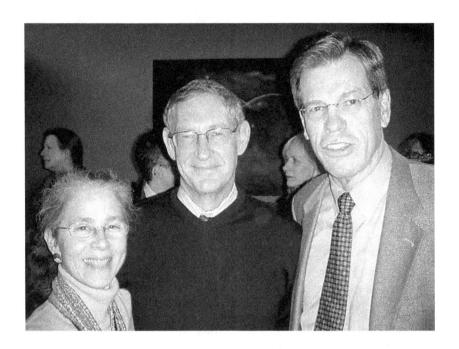

(Top) Judith Wasserheit trained as an ID fellow from 1982–1984 with Holmes and David Eschenbach. Shown here with Larry Corey and Walt Stamm, she led the CDC's Division of STD/HIV Prevention before returning to Seattle in 2001 at Corey's behest to be executive director of the HIV Clinical Trials Network. *Photo courtesy of King Holmes*

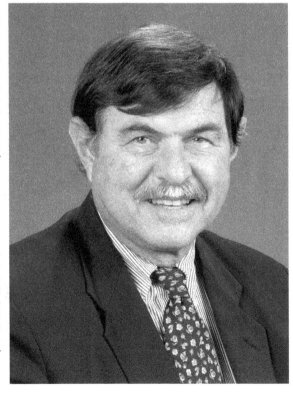

One of Holmes's early fellows, obstetrician-gynecologist David Eschenbach went on to cofound the Infectious Diseases Society for Obstetrics and Gynecology and chair the UW's OB-GYN department. *Photo courtesy of the University of Washington*

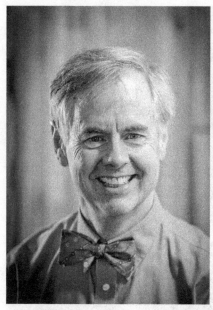
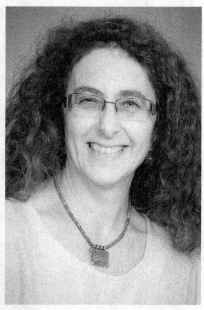

(Left) Wesley Van Voorhis trained as an ID fellow with Klebanoff from 1986–1989; his research focus was the molecular biology of parasites. He became the division's first fellowship director—"The best people from around the country applied for the program," he said—and led the division itself from 2007–2017. *Photo courtesy of the University of Washington*

(Right) Anna Wald was an ID fellow from 1991–1994 with Corey. An expert in herpesviruses, she became director of the UW Virology Research Clinic at Harborview and, in 2017, director of UW's ID division. *Photo courtesy of the University of Washington*

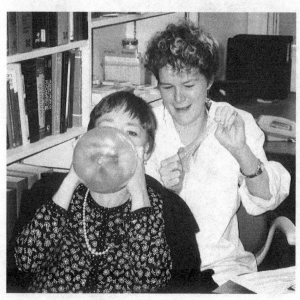

Jeanne Marrazzo, right, was an ID fellow from 1992–1994. A UW faculty member for 21 years, she was medical director of the Seattle STD/HIV Prevention and Training Center and codirector of the STD/AIDS Research Training Fellowship Program. (And yes, those are condoms.) *Photo courtesy of King Holmes*

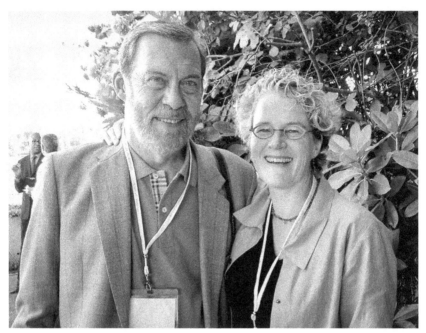

Hunter Handsfield with Jeanne Marrazzo, whom he mentored. An expert on the female vaginal microbiome, Marrazzo succeeded Ned Hook as director of the ID division at the University of Alabama in 2016. *Photo courtesy of H. Hunter Handsfield*

Former fellows developed relationships and networks that endured. Pictured here are Allan Ronald, who was Marvin Turck's first fellow; Sevgi Aral from the CDC's Division of STD Prevention; and Robert Brunham. *Photo by H. Hunter Handsfield*

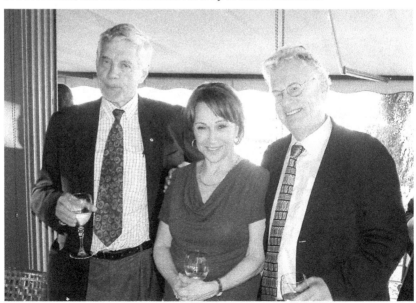

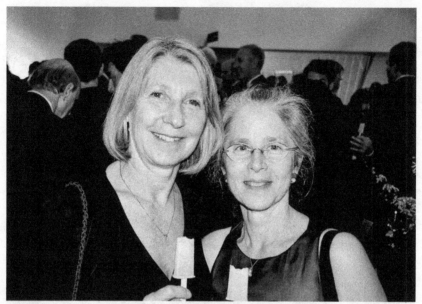

Said Sheila Lukehart of the ID division: "The thing that's changed the most is all the woman." Lukehart, left, took over from King Holmes as director of the UW STD & HIV Research Training Program and served as an associate dean for research and graduate education. Judith Wasserheit, right, succeeded Holmes as director of UW Global Health. *Photo by H. Hunter Handsfield*

Seattle ID researchers and partners—both professional and in real life. Shown from left to right: Connie Celum, Virginia Gonzales, Patricia McInturff, Jo Hoffmann, Jeanne Keruly, Tom Quinn, Jeanne Marrazzo, Linda Summers, and King Holmes. *Photo by H. Hunter Handsfield*

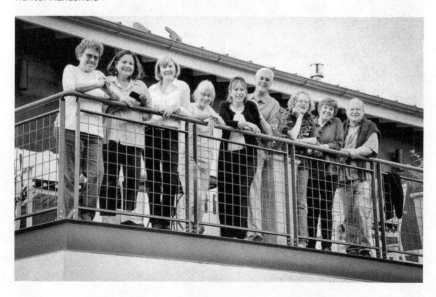

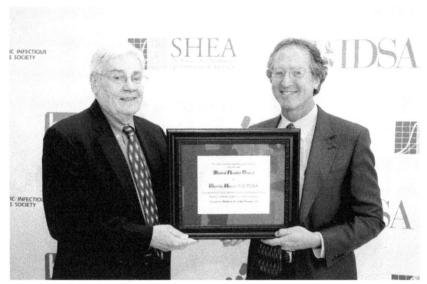

Renowned as a teacher, Marvin Turck, left, received the Infectious Diseases Society of America's Clinical Teaching Award in 2013. The UW Medical School named its Marvin Turck Outstanding Teacher Award in his honor. *Photo courtesy of IDSA*

King Holmes, left, reunited with his first fellows: Paul Wiesner, H. Hunter Handsfield, and Jim Harnisch. *Photo courtesy of King Holmes*

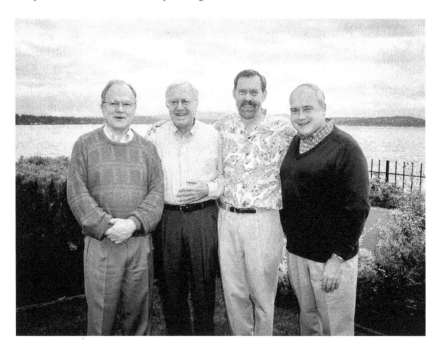

7

AIDS
Changes Everything

The viral pandemic that has now infected more than 75 million people and counting was still in its infancy when Larry Corey called his mentor and colleagues into a meeting and told them, "The infectious disease division needs to own AIDS."[148]

King Holmes, Hunter Handsfield, Walt Stamm, and David Eschenbach agreed.

Although it may seem apparent now, AIDS was not initially the province of infectious-diseases specialists. Oncologists like Paul Volberding of San Francisco General Hospital were among the first to notice the emerging threat when patients began to appear with a cancer, Kaposi sarcoma (KS). The purple skin lesions of KS sent other early patients to dermatologists. General internists were seeing once-healthy people who were losing weight and experiencing mysterious night sweats and infections.

Corey had suspected that a virus was involved ever since that day in June 1981, when, coffee mug in hand, he scanned the latest edition of the MMWR, the CDC's compilation of public health information and alerts. Like physicians and researchers across the world, he read about five previously healthy men, all of them gay, who had fallen ill or died from a lung infection that typically affects only people with severely damaged immune systems. A month later, a second MMWR published an account of 26 patients, all gay, with Kaposi sarcoma or *Pneumocystis carinii* pneumonia (now called *P. jirovecii*).

A self-professed "viral-disease chauvinist," Corey reacted the way he would to any mysterious illness with an unknown cause. "It must be a virus," he thought to himself.[149]

When Hunter Handsfield and ID fellow Ann Collier started seeing gay men with a mysterious lymphadenopathy syndrome showing up at the Seattle–King County STD Clinic, Corey and his lab—acting on his hunch—played around at trying to isolate a virus.

But mostly Corey focused on the work that then commanded most of his attention—developing the drug acyclovir to treat herpes. He had no way of knowing that the MMWR reports would shape the next decades of his career.

In 1983, researchers at the Pasteur Institute in France found the virus—a retrovirus eventually named HIV—behind AIDS. That's when Burroughs Wellcome (now GlaxoSmithKline) turned to Corey, their star on the acyclovir studies. Would he be interested in doing the human studies for a compound that looked promising in laboratory tests against the newly discovered virus?

Then in the midst of writing up and publishing his acyclovir findings, Corey declined. That compound was azidothymidine, or AZT. As it turned out, AZT was only marginally effective, but it started the world down a fast path toward truly effective anti-HIV drugs and treatment.

Later, as the scope of the epidemic became clear, Corey would kick himself for that decision. He and other herpes researchers across the country retooled themselves as HIV researchers. By 1987, he was working 100-hour weeks to lead the NIH-funded AIDS Clinical Trials Group, driven not just by the urgency of the growing epidemic but to make up for having passed up the earlier involvement.

But the time arguably wasn't lost.

To Handsfield, it's impossible to overstate the contribution that Corey's work with acyclovir made toward finding treatments for HIV and other viral diseases. Until acyclovir, Handsfield said, the oft-repeated adage was "You can't treat a virus."

In the 1980s, the field of virology was in its infancy. It wasn't until the 1950s and 1960s that scientists had the tools to understand that these inconceivably tiny pathogens replicate by invading other cells, injecting their genes and proteins and manipulating the host cell into making new copies of the virus. Viruses hijack human genetic machinery in such an integrative way that to interfere with a virus was to interfere with human physiology—the belief was that it just couldn't be done, at least without causing greater harm than good.

Because antiviral treatment was considered such a forlorn hope, Handsfield said, viral diseases were looked on as something of a research black hole. He credits King Holmes for recruiting a researcher to revive that hope. After expanding the focus of STD research beyond syphilis and gonorrhea to include herpes—and later, hepatitis B and human papillomavirus—Holmes knew it was important to bring in a virologist.

And Larry Corey was heretical enough to take up the challenge.

"So King recruits Larry to start the ball rolling in terms of virologic STDs, mainly herpes," said Handsfield. "Well, that explodes. Acyclovir is the first effective, non-toxic treatment for a viral infection. That treatment for an STD becomes the nexus for all the growth that happened since, regarding everything from oseltamivir—Tamiflu—for influenza to the panoply of drugs for HIV to hepatitis C, hepatitis B, and a whole number of other viral diseases. The start of national recognition of virology as a clinically productive area that has therapeutic value as well as intellectual value was largely centered here."[150]

But as far as treating this new sexually transmitted viral disease was concerned, there would be dark days to get through first.

Serving Seattle: Hunter Handsfield and Ann Collier

Early on in the epidemic, from 1982 to 1985, Handsfield and a newly arrived infectious-diseases fellow, Ann Collier, became the faces of Seattle's public health response to AIDS.

Handsfield already had expanded the Seattle–King County public health STD program to include emerging STIs. What was to prove equally important, he had developed a strong relationship with community groups at high risk of such infections, including men who have sex with men, building on work begun when he was one of King Holmes's early fellows.

"There had come to be an understanding that the public health department was not a bunch of sex cops, that we were there to provide holistic care," said Handsfield. "That joint public health–academic institutional collaboration plus strong community relationships with high-risk groups meant the rapid growth of what certainly in the early days—and many would say even today—is one of the best HIV/AIDS treatment and prevention programs in the country."[151]

Handsfield's fellow, Ann Collier, would prove instrumental to that program.

A Dartmouth Medical School graduate, Collier was chief medical resident at Dartmouth-Hitchcock Medical Center in 1981 when she saw her first AIDS patient: a young gay man who had moved back home to New Hampshire after falling ill in San Francisco. The still-unnamed syndrome had only just been reported in the MMWR, and Collier assumed she would never see another case.

Instead, AIDS become her life's work.

That same year, she decided that she wanted to pursue training in infectious diseases, but she had not applied to any fellowship programs. When she saw an ad in the *New England Journal of Medicine* for an unexpected ID fellowship opening at the University of Washington, she said to herself, "That's got my name on it."

She arrived in Seattle in July 1982, the month the city reported its first AIDS diagnosis. Collier's first meeting with King Holmes was memorable in part because of the two other new fellows—Judith Wasserheit and Anne Rompalo—she met while they all waited for their (late-running) appointments outside Holmes's office. The trio would become lifelong friends and infectious-diseases research leaders.

Offered a choice of projects, Collier went to work with Handsfield on an NIH-funded grant related to cytomegalovirus (CMV). Hypothesizing that CMV might be a cause or contributor to AIDS (it was not), Handsfield, with NIH approval, had parlayed the study into a broader investigation into persistent generalized lymphadenopathy. He had begun seeing gay men in the STD clinic with swollen lymph nodes in more than one part of the body that lasted for more than a couple of weeks—a condition that had piqued Corey's attention as well.

Collier found in Handsfield a supportive mentor who, in the "off you go!" ethos of the division, delegated readily. As she began enrolling patients in their cohort study comparing men with generalized lymphadenopathy to those without, word got out in the larger gay community. The phones began ringing with people wanting to be in the study.

"This was incredibly dramatic," she said. "All of a sudden there were hundreds in my study with this condition, who were previously healthy, relatively young, mostly gay men in an era where AIDS was being described."[152]

Handsfield and Collier did their best to address the rising fear.

"We had community meetings with 300 or 400 people—if the fire marshal had come around, they would have kicked us out," Handsfield recalled. "We were continually and routinely available on request to meet with groups and talk with them."[153]

The connection between lymphadenopathy and the newly identified syndrome was later confirmed, as was the new disease's rapid spread. Once HIV was identified as the virus behind AIDS in 1984 and a test developed to detect it in 1985, the researchers tested the samples that they had collected during their study. Ninety-nine percent of the people with persistent general lymphadenopathy had HIV antibodies—as did 30 percent of the supposedly healthy controls.

When her fellowship ended, Collier followed in Ned Hooks's footsteps to become assistant director of the STD clinic. But the STD clinic wasn't set up to provide continuing care, and that's what the men in her study increasingly needed as AIDS took its toll. As the number of infections rose, so did pressure to learn how to handle this frightening disease. Collier stepped up, learning as she went.

"So that's how I became an AIDS doctor," Collier said. "No one knew anything about it at all. I didn't know much, but I knew more than anybody else."

"We didn't know how big the iceberg was"

Robert Wood—"Dr. Bob" to his patients and the public—also didn't know anything about AIDS when he was asked to care for one of the first people to be diagnosed in Seattle.

"I'm not an ID doc, but I sort of played an ID doc," he said. "Because I'm a gay man, I got recruited to take care of one of the first AIDS cases in the region in late 1982."[154]

Born in Elmira, New York, Wood received his MD at the University of Rochester in 1970 and trained in internal medicine at Dartmouth-Hitchcock Hospitals. He was a commissioned officer of the US Navy from 1972 to 1974, then returned to Dartmouth as a Fellow in Health Services Research. After joining the Public Health Service, he arrived in Seattle in 1975 as director of research at the US Public Health Hospital; in 1977, he became an assistant professor of medicine at the UW. His research focused on developing computer algorithms to predict common clinical problems and develop standards of care.

In the late 1970s, Wood began volunteering at the newly opened Seattle Gay Clinic. He also helped organize a group of fellow LGBTQ, or lesbian, gay, bisexual, transgender, and queer (or questioning) physicians who shared his interest in the health care needs of gays and lesbians. Little did the physicians know then what was coming.

Early in 1982—barely six months after the first cases of what was not yet named AIDS had been reported—one of Wood's friends complained of having night sweats and bumps all over his body. Suspecting Hodgkin's disease or lymphoma, Wood arranged for his friend to be seen at the Public Health Hospital and to have a lymph node biopsied. He and King Holmes, who was then chief of infectious diseases at that hospital, later peered at the sample under the microscope and concluded that the friend was suffering the same generalized lymphadenopathy that Handsfield and Collier were studying and that was later recognized as an early sign of AIDS.

Holmes had a way of pulling bright researchers into his orbit. Wood became one of them.

"King knew that I was a gay man," Wood said. "He would let me read some of the papers he and his fellows were writing. Sometimes I would give King and others feedback on how they were thinking about gay people. He was always very receptive."

While Wood knew that attitudes and biases toward LGBTQ people were "just ensconced in the social fabric," the straight infectious-diseases physicians and researchers he worked with were, he said, for the most part nonjudgmental.

"King has a great, open mind," Wood said. "He is so pragmatic and into science, I don't think he has much room for biases about sexual orientation."

Wood in turn found himself learning about infectious diseases and epidemiology, not just from Holmes but from other luminaries around him, including Marvin Turck and Walt Stamm, whose lectures he sought out.

Later in 1982, Wood, again at the request of friends, took on the care of one of King County's earliest cases of AIDS, which by then had a name. The patient had come down with pneumocystis pneumonia in Hawaii and was treated for it in San Francisco. But by the time the man arrived in Seattle, he had fevers, night sweats, and had acquired another opportunistic infection, which required CDC-authorized drugs and a brief hospitalization. Shortly after his release, the man returned to his family home in Ohio, where he died.

"It was pretty scary in those early days," Wood said. "We didn't know how big the iceberg was, but we were seeing only the tip of it in cases of AIDS."[155]

The Madison Clinic and AIDS prevention

Around this time, Joan Kreiss, another fellow of Holmes's, returned from working with Allan Ronald in Kenya, where she was among the first to recognize the toll that AIDS was taking among female sex workers. Kreiss understood what was coming and joined Collier in pressing to start a Seattle clinic, separate from the STD clinic, that was solely for people with HIV and included primary care.

Harborview Medical Center became one of the first hospitals in the country to open such a clinic—first a small one and then, in 1985, the larger Madison Clinic, cofounded by Collier and Kreiss, on the corner of Broadway and Madison. (It later moved to the west clinic wing of Harborview, but the name remains.) The Madison Clinic, according to Handsfield, is an outstanding example of what could be accomplished by the "Seattle model"—the cooperative relationship that Holmes and his early fellows had begun building in the late 1970s with the Seattle–King County Department of Public Health.

Bob Wood, whose AIDS case numbers were increasing at the US Public Health Hospital, decided to transfer his patients to the new clinic as soon as it was established. "Basically, a bunch of us had the idea that if we put all the AIDS/HIV patients together, we'd learn from each other what we were seeing," he said.

The public health department worked closely with the university and Harborview to find funding and space and build support in both the gay and the wider communities. The clinic's creation was all the more impressive considering the stigma and fear that surrounded AIDS at that time, which was reflected in naming the clinic for its location rather than its specialty.

Holmes, by then chief of medicine at Harborview, lent his support, as did Patricia McInturff, the public health department's section administrator for STDs and the department's liaison to the county-appointed Harborview trustees.

In addition, McInturff assembled a community advisory group to find funding for outreach and prevention. In much of the rest of the country, different factions competed for AIDS resources. Seattle stood out for its cooperation among public health, academia, and community. The public health department won a grant from the CDC to run one of the nation's first AIDS demonstration projects, under Wood's direction, followed by a significant grant from the Robert Wood Johnson Foundation to fund coordination of AIDS services.

"We had the scientists behind us, the university researchers, the community," said McInturff, who is married to Handsfield. "The people who came together around this were some of the smartest, most dedicated people I've ever worked with."[156]

Wood was one of them. He was already a member of the advisory group when Handsfield asked him to be medical director of the Seattle–King County AIDS Control Program. Wood liked working on complex medical problems, and he liked working with Handsfield and McInturff. But there was another reason the job felt like the right fit: in May 1985, around the time testing first became available, Wood learned that he was HIV positive.

Ann Collier gave him the test results. He went sailing in Greece for five weeks to process the information, then returned to Handsfield's job offer.

"Here I am, I'm HIV-positive, maybe I'm going to die of AIDS," Wood said. "But I can bring some of my skills to helping bring this under control and take care of people while I'm in the process of dying and do some good on this problem that infects mostly gay men." He started his new job in 1986.

Wood didn't wait for those at risk to come into a clinic. Candid about his own status, he reached out, whether in speaking to community groups or writing his "Dr. Bob" column for the local gay paper. He didn't shy from controversy either. He supported one of the country's first needle exchange programs in Tacoma. He backed a state AIDS reporting regulation over protests by gay groups. And he encouraged testing for HIV at a time many didn't want to endure the anxiety and stigma for a diagnosis that had no treatment.

Testing told him who to worry about, he said. And if HIV itself could not be treated, Wood argued that progress was being made on treating the opportunistic infections it gave rise to, some of which could be prevented prophylactically.[157] He also counseled those who tested positive on how not to transmit HIV, "deputizing" them, as the AIDS Control officer, to help him rein in the epidemic that had become the No. 1 killer of young men from ages 25 to 44.

In those early days, before life-saving treatments were developed, the urgency of the mission was underscored by the number of funerals the group attended, a searing memory even decades later.

Not surprisingly, the STD and HIV research and prevention programs attracted many bright, determined gay men to positions throughout the public health and UW medicine communities. To witness some of these health educators, counselors, care providers, and administrators became ill with AIDS and die was both motivating and devastating.

"You don't usually start going to funerals in your life for people your own age—37-, 38-, 39-years-old," McInturff said.[158]

Her administrative leadership of the nascent public health HIV/AIDS program led to McInturff being recognized in 1992 with the first Washington State Governors AIDS Service Award for Public Service, yet another award for a de facto trainee and revered colleague of the UW programs.[159]

Wood went on to become nationally recognized for his research and prevention work and to serve on the CDC HIV/STD advisory committee. The Seattle–King County AIDS program served as a model for public health agencies across the country, with Wood twice invited to present the program's methods and findings at WHO meetings in Geneva, in 1987 and again in 1998.

Collier also recalled her work in those early years as "intellectually incredibly interesting and emotionally very challenging." As she followed her study enrollees over time, many of them died. Some referred partners and friends to her for the study, and they died too. The clinic could offer supportive care and a social worker and, eventually, treat or prevent some opportunistic infections, like pneumocystis. But other opportunistic infections would come along and cause death regardless.

Seeing so many deaths compelled her toward treatment research. When the NIH put out a call for grants, Collier already met one of its requirements—a cohort of patients with HIV. She needed someone who knew how to grow the virus in the lab.

She went to Larry Corey.

The ACTG and the search for treatments

Corey was already thinking along the same lines.

"As a field, infectious diseases needs to start embracing this," he had told Holmes, Handsfield, Stamm, and Eschenbach in that early meeting. "We should build out a clinic that can be both a research and a clinical care clinic. We need to learn how to take care of people and develop therapies."[160]

Together with Joel Meyers's work with infections in transplant patients at Fred Hutch, Corey had already established Seattle as a strong virology research center. Now he sent a new ID fellow—Canadian Robert Coombs, a physician and microbiologist—to learn from Harvard virologist Martin S. Hirsch how to isolate HIV. When Coombs returned, Corey lobbied for the UW Medical Center campus to open a lab for him, although HIV clinical care remained at Harborview.

Over Christmas break 1985, Corey sat down in his office with Collier to write the grant. They got it, with Corey the principal investigator and Collier the director of the UW AIDS Clinical Trial Unit.

The UW unit became part of a network named the AIDS Clinical Trials Group, or ACTG, with units based at top academic institutions throughout the country. Although such units were common in the cancer field, "There was no precedent for the ultimate magnitude of this [undertaking]," said Dr. Anthony Fauci, who became director of the National Institute of Allergy and Infectious Diseases (NIAID) in 1984. Creating a network of these units, Fauci said, would allow pooling of data and deliver answers more quickly.

"We were dealing with a disease that was essentially 100 percent fatal," he said in an interview marking the 30th anniversary of AIDS. "So when we were trying to determine whether a drug worked or not, we needed to know the answer right away."[161]

The person tapped to be chair of the executive committee overseeing this precedent-setting undertaking was Corey. He was not yet 40 years old when he undertook the most ambitious program of his career to date, but his ability to skate to where the puck was going had been there ever since he was made the administrator of his Jewish summer camp as a teenager. He seemed to just intuitively know, "This is what should happen." The structure that he set up for the ACTG in 1986 is still in place today.

Corey's work on acyclovir had already made him one of the most consulted virologists in the country. But with the new appointment, he said, "My life changed a lot."[162]

With no budget for hotel stays, he would catch a red-eye flight in the early morning from Seattle to Washington DC to attend meetings at NIH headquarters in Bethesda, Maryland, returning home on the day's last flight. So urgent was the need for therapies that study investigators routinely worked seven-day, 100-hour weeks.

Corey knew the urgency firsthand. Every year, he would invite someone with AIDS to speak to the virology class he taught for first-year medical students. In those still-early days before treatments, even some healthcare workers were afraid to be in the same room with AIDS patients. Corey wanted to make sure that his students didn't buy into that fear.

"I would break the class up into small groups and they would have some one-on-one with the person about what it was like to have AIDS," he said. "They would see me shake hands with the person and hug the person. There's a humanity aspect to this."[163]

What hit Corey hardest—the real "humanity aspect"—was that each year, he had to recruit new patients.

"The patients I brought in to be with the class one year were never around the next year," he said. "They all died before you could bring them back. Every single one."[164]

As the public face of the network overseeing clinical trials of HIV treatment, Corey would bear the rage, frustration, and grief of a community being ravaged by those deaths.

As the network was being organized, Burroughs Wellcome came out with its study showing AZT extended life in people with full-blown AIDS. The first trials built off that discovery. But soon activists began protesting against AZT because of its perceived toxicity.

The AIDS activist group ACT UP dubbed Corey and ACTG investigators Margaret Fischl of the University of Miami, Martin S. Hirsch of Harvard, Thomas Merigan of Stanford, and Douglas Richman of the University of California at San Diego the "Gang of Five" and publicly accused them of "ignoring the anger and frustration of people whose lives are at stake." In a mock trial on the streets of San Francisco, activists tried the five scientists for "their crimes against gay people."

Anthony Fauci scolded the activists in the pages of the *Advocate* newspaper, saying, "It is particularly devastating and unfair when scientists of good faith and enormous talent are singled out and publicly named as scoundrels."

Fauci later suggested that community members be allowed to attend the ACTG's meetings. By the end of 1990, each site sought the local community's involvement when developing studies. Today, community advisory boards are the norm in HIV research and a model for other disease advocates.

Corey today is one of the staunchest advocates of patient and community involvement, but the bitterness of the protests took their toll. He tried to hold on to a lesson that his beloved brother-in-law, whose death spurred Corey to specialize in infectious diseases, taught him—that to be educated was to be tolerant.

"You sometimes have to have the maturity of age to step back and say, 'Well, OK, you could have handled that better,'" he said. "There is some wisdom that comes out of parts of your life where you get criticized. You learn from your experience."

He never lost his focus on the goal. As head of the executive committee, he was the person behind the scenes who defined the priorities of the ACTG and facilitated the rapid move from single- to double- to triple-combination therapy. Bob Coombs's first major article—after returning from the Hirsch lab—showed that HIV could readily be isolated from the blood of Ann Colliers's patients with lymphadenopathy syndrome. It set the principle for early therapy and an important ACTG study call ACG 116 that Corey designed with

Paul Volberding of San Francisco General. Corey was particularly proud of a study that showed AZT could prevent mother-to-child transmission, a finding made after he sidestepped the protestors by forming a separate pediatric arm for the research group.[165]

The ACTG developed and tested combination drug therapies and then protease inhibitors that by 1996 extended the life of people with HIV from between 6 and 9 months to 20 years. Today, those who have access to treatment—Bob Wood among them—can live a near-normal lifespan.

"I think it's the most remarkable achievement in all of medicine," Corey said. "Just look at the number of lives saved, the number of young adults who are living."

HIV research goes global

With Corey and Collier leading national efforts to find treatment and Handsfield and Wood leading the local response, King Holmes looked toward international efforts.

Canadian Allan Ronald—Marvin Turck's first fellow who was now at the University of Manitoba—had begun a research collaboration with the University of Nairobi in 1978 after Kenyan microbiologist Herbert Nsanze had contacted him about his work on a chancroid outbreak in Winnipeg.

Once in Nairobi, Ronald noticed that, in addition to chancroid, other STIs such as gonorrhea and chlamydia also were rampant. Ronald brought in his fellow, Frank Plummer, to broaden the research program. He also turned for advice to Holmes, whom he knew slightly from his UW days and by reputation as the leading expert on research into STIs. Holmes sent a fellow of his with interests in epidemiology and international research—Joan Kreiss, who would later help Collier open the Madison Clinic—to Nairobi in 1984.

The researchers noted that many men seeking treatment at government clinics had frequented sex workers in a Nairobi slum. The team enrolled a cohort of sex workers in a study to measure the prevalence of STDs.

Kreiss had been a student at California State University when the first US AIDS cases were identified. She wanted to test the female sex workers in Nairobi for HIV. Ronald and Holmes tried to talk her out of it. There were scant reports of HIV in Eastern Africa, and the people most at risk of contracting HIV in the United States and Europe were men who had sex with men or hemophiliacs and injection drug users.

Kreiss persisted. And to the team's astonishment, two out of three women tested were positive for HIV.

"Joan Kreiss was a major help in sorting out the epidemiology of HIV," Ronald said.

Kreiss published her findings in the *New England Journal of Medicine* in 1986. Given the fear and stigma surrounding HIV, the resulting furor nearly drove Ronald and Plummer out of Kenya. Their Kenyan colleagues rallied to their defense.

By 1988 the University of Washington formally became a collaborating institution.

"King made a huge difference," Ronald said. "He sort of took over the program almost. He had NIH resources and was a brilliant ID man. He became very much the guru that everybody went to."[166]

In 1988, Holmes and Kreiss started the UW International AIDS Research and Training Program focusing on training researchers in Kenya, Peru, Mozambique, and Thailand. Kreiss continued to do research in Kenya, launching a study of perinatal HIV transmission. Virologist Julie Overbaugh, a UW professor of microbiology based at Fred Hutch, joined the project in the early 1990s and established a base in Mombasa, Kenya.

The Mombasa Cohort, continued by Overbaugh after Kreiss left science, has become the longest continuously running African cohort aimed at assessing risk of HIV infection.[167] In addition to important findings on intervention and prevention, it has been a training site for a new generation of HIV researchers such as UW's Jared Baeten, who would later lead large studies showing the efficacy of pre-exposure prophylaxis, or PrEP, and the dapivirine vaginal ring against HIV transmission.

The Nairobi-based Kenyan program also continued to make seminal contributions, including being the first to show that male circumcision may lower the risk of HIV infection.

Peter Piot, too, played a significant role in addressing HIV/AIDS globally, as did other former UW fellows from Holmes's orbit. Piot began working in Kenya with Allan Ronald and Herbert Nsanze in

Kenya in 1981, just as the first cases were being reported in the United States.

Before HIV had yet been identified as the cause of AIDS, Piot and former Holmes fellow Tom Quinn convinced the NIH in 1983 to send them to Kinshasa, Zaire (now the Democratic Republic of Congo), to investigate whether a life-threatening illness known as "slim disease" was the same as AIDS.

An analysis of medical records showed that the wasting and opportunistic infections that characterized AIDS had been present in Central Africa since at least the 1970s, which was later confirmed when a test for the virus was developed and applied to stored blood samples.

"This was the beginning of an extremely productive period of research, mainly in Zaire and Kenya, that gave us a wealth of basic knowledge about HIV/AIDS in sub-Saharan Africa," Piot said. Armed with that knowledge, Piot in 1995 became the founding executive director of UNAIDS.[168] Quinn went on to serve as a senior investigator at NIAID and head of its section on international HIV/STD research, investigating HIV/AIDS in more than 26 countries. Both scientists continued to work with Holmes, Corey, Handsfield, Collier, Judy Wasserheit, and other Seattle-based or trained infectious-diseases researchers throughout their careers.

That Seattle network, Piot said, became an integral part of HIV research.

"It was the whole infrastructure—not bricks and mortar, but the kind of attitude and discipline needed to deal with HIV," he said. "It had a very strong clinical component, epidemiology, a well-functioning STD clinic. And also, King's intellectual curiosity driving us all to be at the forefront of new things."[169]

Holmes expanded his international involvement, forging relationships in Lima through Jorge Sanchez, an infectious-diseases specialist who came to Seattle for a master's in public health and returned to direct the Peruvian HIV control program. King helped found the UW Center for AIDS and STDs in 1989, which became one of the first in the US to shift much of its research focus to AIDS in the developing world, and started a second training program, the International Training and Education Center for Health, which trains thousands of workers in 30 countries to do clinical and laboratory work on HIV. He worked with Allan Ronald and AIDS researcher Merle Sande—who had once counseled a young Ned Hook to pursue infectious-diseases research—to train health workers at the Infectious Diseases Institute that Ronald and Sande helped create in Kampala, Uganda.

"He picked up the international health mantel over HIV," said Corey, crediting his mentor for "incredible vision" for doing so.

It was not called "global health" yet. But soon, it would be. And Corey, too, would play a role, going from HIV treatment to heading a new global network to pursue an even more challenging goal—an HIV vaccine.

How HIV changed infectious diseases

HIV did more than help birth global health. It also changed the field of infectious diseases itself. Although those physician-researchers who focused on STDs were used to seeing patients in outpatient clinics, many other ID specialists worked in hospitals or with surgeons to treat or prevent infections. Maybe they ran a micro-lab.

HIV was the first real outpatient infectious disease. Before, every infection was acute—a patient got better, or they died. End of story. No one really took care of such patients over the long term.

"HIV changed that," said Corey. "It created a private practice in infectious diseases. It created enormous numbers of ID people."[170]

The response to AIDS had lasting impact, beyond infectious diseases. It provided a model of collaboration, not just between researchers and clinicians but among nurses, patients, and communities. Especially in those dark early years before treatment, it forced national conversations on end-of-life care. It even changed cultural mores inside and outside medicine, shifting the way people regard sexual orientation.

"I never thought as a gay man that I would see gay marriage accepted as a right by the Supreme Court," said Bob Wood. "AIDS brought LGBT issues to the forefront. If we had all stayed in the closet and died, AIDS wouldn't have created that change."[171]

The AIDS pandemic also reminded a complacent public—including other physician-scientists—that infectious diseases weren't over.

The antibiotic revolution that made it possible to actually cure many infectious diseases had in some ways created the new subspecialty in internal medicine, attracting more physicians and spawning infectious-diseases divisions in medical schools and fellowship programs to meet the growing interest. The American Medical Association established board certification for infectious diseases in 1974; Hunter Handsfield was in the first group to take the exam.

Then, almost as soon as it was formally recognized, people began questioning whether the subspecialty was still needed. Petersdorf was hardly alone in his earlier thinking that better sanitation, antibiotics, and vaccines had all but conquered infectious diseases.

HIV would shatter that notion. That MMWR report on June 5, 1981, was reported in only a handful of newspapers. But soon it became one of the most heavily quoted articles in the medical literature. HIV/AIDS would change not just how medical and public health experts worked together to prevent and control infectious diseases but how they looked for emerging infections to thwart the next pandemic.

And there would be a next time.

When John Sherris, the pioneering microbiology chairman who had helped train Corey and other early UW infectious-diseases fellows, retired in 1986, he gave a final lecture on the flu epidemic that swept the world in 1918, killing at least 50 million people.

"We're seeing evidence of new viruses cropping up in different parts of the world, causing all sorts of trouble," he said. "It will be amazing if we are not hit dramatically by something that would make the 1918 influenza epidemic look like a ride in the park. We live in a fool's paradise. The bugs are going to get us in the end."[172]

8

A Diverse Portfolio
of Research

A IDS transformed and dominated infectious diseases through the 1980s and 1990s. But while many Seattle infectious-diseases physician-researchers redirected their careers to pursue the pathogen—a signature strength of the division was how nimbly it pivoted to new challenges—not everyone focused solely on HIV.

Joel Meyers spent the 1980s launching the first program in the country to study and treat the unique infections that plague bone marrow transplant patients. George Counts moved from serving as chief of infectious diseases at Harborview to working with Meyers at Fred Hutch as head of its microbiology program and laboratory. And Jim Harnisch made Seattle into an unlikely hub of leprosy research.

Two new fellows arrived who would go on to become the next generation of builders—King Holmes's mentee Judith Wasserheit, who worked with David Eschenbach on STIs as they affect women's and children's health, and Klebanoff's mentee Wes Van Voorhis, whose passion was parasitology.

The guiding light

Joel Meyers had first met transplantation pioneer E. Donnall Thomas in 1974 when Meyers was dispatched by the EIS to investigate an outbreak of what turned out to be hepatitis C in the UW transplant ward at the Public Health Service Hospital. That had sparked his interest in the infectious complications of transplant patients and drew him back to Seattle, along with EIS colleagues and lifelong friends Larry Corey and Walt Stamm.

After completing an infectious-diseases fellowship, Meyers received a UW School of Medicine faculty appointment in 1978 and formally joined Fred Hutch, Thomas's new home, then located on Seattle's First Hill.

Both Meyers and Corey were "bright people who contributed to our understanding of viruses themselves and of viral infections, at a time when our understanding of viruses was limited," said Jim Harnisch.[173]

Thomas and Meyers wrote a grant to support Meyers and the development of an in-house infectious diseases program,[174] the first such program in the country, which Meyers was named to head in 1982. The academic research program would touch on all of the predominant infectious-diseases problems in marrow transplant recipients, studying the epidemiology and pathogenesis of viruses, bacteria and molds, improving their diagnoses, and developing treatments.

But Meyers would have just a decade to build the program before he died of colon cancer.

He zeroed in on cytomegalovirus, or CMV, a type of herpesvirus, confirming that it was indeed the leading infectious killer of transplant patients and not just a casual bystander, with a fatality rate for CMV pneumonia approaching 90 percent.

"Not only did he define that CMV was a pathogen, he did the first studies to show that he could treat that pathogen and almost make it go away," Corey said. "Being able to discover it and then treat it, in such a short period of time—it was cool that he got to see that, he got to know that, before his premature death."[175]

Among Meyers's boldest studies, according to Corey, were clinical trials that showed that treating bone marrow transplant patients prophylactically with antibiotics or antivirals saved lives by *preventing* deadly infections. One of those studies showed that the antiviral drug ganciclovir, a close relative of acyclovir, could prevent deaths from CMV.

The discovery revolutionized bone marrow transplantation. Because of the risk of infection, patients undergoing bone marrow transplants used to be hospitalized for 100 days in isolated, sterile environments with controlled air flow and irradiated food. Today, many stem cell transplants take place on an outpatient basis with antibiotics or antivirals used prophylactically to prevent infections.

When Don Thomas received the Nobel Prize in 1990, Meyers was among those he acknowledged as having made "major contributions to the achievements honored by this award."[176]

In the early days of transplantation, "infection was the most common cause of death in patients with bone marrow transplantation as well as those undergoing cancer chemotherapy," said Dr. Philip Pizzo, a former Stanford medical school dean and an expert in infectious diseases and pediatric blood cancers who authored several papers with Meyers. "That has changed. And it has changed because of people like Joel."[177]

Using such strong drugs prophylactically had been considered heretical at the time. Pizzo and others who have followed in Meyers's footsteps now refer to the "Joel Meyers dictum": prevention is usually more successful than treatment and often much less expensive.

"In the 1980s, everyone thought the Hutch [researchers] were the cowboys," said James C. Wade, Meyers's first trainee, who went on to become deputy director of quality, clinical operations, and network development at the Virginia-based Inova Schar Cancer Institute. "They were out doing the wild things. They were the ones who were blazing what would be the future."[178]

When Meyers was diagnosed with advanced colon cancer, Wade helped him and his wife, Barbara Thrasher-Meyers, make tough treatment decisions. As a last-ditch effort, Meyers underwent an experimental bone marrow transplant himself.[179] It did not work against the cancer.

He died in October 1991, weeks before his ganciclovir study was published in the *New England Journal of Medicine*. He was 46 years old.

Corey organized the memorial service. At Thrasher's request, he, Walt Stamm, and Lucy Tompkins delivered eulogies.

Twenty-five year later, Corey, Tompkins, and others remembered Meyers at a symposium to honor his legacy.

"He defined what a program should do: Recognize problems. Study them systematically. Take care of people," said Corey, who also recalled how good Meyers was at building trust between infectious-diseases physicians and oncologists. Immunologist Stan Riddell recalled Meyers as "a gentleman in dress and demeanor."

"I never heard Joel say anything bad about anybody," Tompkins said. "But he had this wicked wit. That wry little smile of Joel's—I'll always remember him that way."[180]

The symposium—on infectious diseases in the immunocompromised host—drew about 150 luminaries in the now-established field, including a dozen researchers whose early work was funded by an endowment scholarship named for Meyers. Barbara Thrasher and her second husband, Rick Koffey, fund the scholarship, established with Corey's help and the support of Michael Boeckh, who came to Seattle as an infectious-diseases fellow in 1990 to train with Meyers and now heads the Hutch's Infectious Disease Sciences Program.

Meyers's death left Boeckh with the feeling that he needed to carry on the work, both in CMV research, in which he has become a leader, and in training others.

"Joel was an iconic leader and inspiring mentor and role model," he said.[181] The mission of the Joel Meyers Endowment Scholarship is to create leaders, and it has, with recipients going on to head the Transplant and Oncology Program at Johns Hopkins University School of Medicine, lead epidemiology and prevention at the CDC, and serve as chief medical officers at biomedicine companies.

George Counts, who as head of the Hutch's microbiology laboratory in the 1980s freed Meyers to focus on virology, recalled his colleague's dedication to his field and to his fellows.

"There are so many good people throughout this ID program, and Joel was one of them," Counts said. "He was a great virologist, he and Larry. Joel was also a good administrator. His fellows loved him, and he was supportive and compassionate towards them."[182]

Added Tompkins, "It's sad that [Joel's] not here today to see the massive explosion of the field that he started and this preeminent program, which is still the guiding light for all of us."[183]

The trailblazer

Marvin Turck had convinced George Counts to return to Seattle in 1975 after five years as an assistant professor of medicine and pathology at the University of Miami. Turck, who had first recruited Counts to Seattle for an infectious-diseases fellowship, lured him back to take a faculty position at the University of Washington and to replace the departing Harry Beaty—the mentor under whom Counts had trained—as chief of infectious diseases at Harborview.

At first, Counts hesitated. His time in Miami had been professionally satisfying, especially his growing involvement in hospital-associated infections and infection control. Yet, despite his success, he worried whether he was up to the challenge Turck posed.

"I wasn't convinced I was good enough to succeed in this high-powered, research-intensive role that the University of Washington ID division practiced," he said. "The program here was so deep in terms of the number of people involved, the basic research, the fact that it was nationally known. It was just a big behemoth, one of the top three or four in the country."[184]

But he had loved his time at Harborview. And he had loved working with Turck, who was entirely convinced he would succeed.

Lucy Tompkins, who was finishing up her residency at Harborview around the time Counts became ID chief, was one of the fellows Counts mentored. She described him as especially supportive, maybe because her experience echoed his. If Tompkins had found it isolating to be a rare female fellow in a mostly male division, Counts had even fewer African-American role models.

He found a lifelong mentor outside the division in Dr. Alvin Thompson, a gastroenterologist at the Seattle Veterans hospital and a clinical professor at the UW Medical School. A Washington DC native, Thompson received his medical degree from Howard University in 1946. Determined to escape the segregation he experienced in his hometown, he moved across the country to Seattle in 1953. He worked tirelessly to help other people of color overcome discrimination, especially in receiving healthcare or training to deliver it.

At the same time, Thompson counseled Counts to focus first on his own career. One of the pressures of being one of very few black faculty members was constantly being asked to serve on a committee or attend an event promoting diversity. Counts found it hard to say no because it was something that he *wanted* to do. "For folks like myself, who came from such desperate backgrounds and had been helped along the way, it's an opportunity to give back," he said.

But Thompson reminded him that he first needed to accomplish the research and publications required to be promoted to full professor, and *then* he could give back.

"He made sure I kept my nose to the grindstone—this is 'publish or perish,'" Counts said. "I have used that as I have interacted with young black faculty members coming along here, both at the fellow level and at the junior faculty level, trying to keep them focused on what they need to do to succeed."

Counts collaborated with both Turck and Walt Stamm on research in UTIs. With Turck, he also worked closely with pharmaceutical companies to test antibiotics.

"One of the things I learned about Marv was his integrity," Counts said of those years. "Many established ID specialists were too closely associated with pharmaceutical companies and ended up serving as consultants. Marv never compromised his relationships. That's one of the things I most admired about him."

Counts continued his research focus on hospital-associated infections, and he was active in the formation of the Association for Professionals in Infection Control and Epidemiology (APIC), becoming its national president in 1983. In 1985, he guided publication of a seminal position paper, "Listen to the Music," calling on the infectious disease community to clearly define the role of infection prevention practitioners.[185]

During this period, he regularly served as attending physician two to three months each year at Fred Hutch, then located in a facility on Seattle's First Hill.

He achieved his goal of becoming a full professor in 1985. That year, he moved to the Hutch full time to direct its clinical microbiology program and laboratory and, along with Joel Meyers, research infections in immune-compromised patients.

And Counts did give back, as his former mentor had assured him that he would. At a time when African-American physicians were largely underrepresented in academic medicine in general and infectious diseases in particular, Counts organized a key networking group for minority ID medical school fellows and faculty within the Infectious Diseases Society of America (IDSA).

"In addition to his stellar accomplishments in research, patient care and teaching, Dr. Counts will be best celebrated for his service as an extraordinary mentor," members of the George W. Counts Interest Group wrote of him. "He was the first minority role model for many of us who attended IDSA annual meetings ... During subsequent years and to this day, the organization founded by Dr. Counts has provided a vehicle for career advancement of minorities within IDSA and has indirectly increased the awareness of health disparities within IDSA and, importantly, in the communities which we serve nationally and globally." [186]

Counts continued these efforts after he left the Hutch in 1989 for NIAID in Bethesda, Maryland, to direct its newly established Clinical Research Management branch. CRUM, as the branch became known, provided logistical support for the urgently needed AIDS treatment trials then getting underway, including those chaired by Larry Corey. Frustrated by what he saw as inadequate recruitment of women and people of color into research studies, Counts also established and directed the Office of Research on Minority and Women's Health. Then he spent two years at the CDC as coordinator of its Plan to Eliminate Syphilis, where his interest in bioethics led him to delve into the Tuskegee syphilis study and its toxic legacy of distrust.

It was perfect preparation for his next position. In 2002, Corey lured Counts back to Seattle to advise the HIV Vaccine Trials Network. Corey saw Counts's experience and stature as key to recruiting and involving the traditionally underserved populations hardest hit by AIDS.

"An incredible and fascinating disease"

As a dermatologist also trained in infectious diseases, Jim Harnisch saw some of the early HIV patients with the skin lesions of Kaposi sarcoma. It was before the virus behind this and a raft of mysterious infections had been identified as HIV.

"Kaposi was almost never seen before HIV," he said. "I knew what it was, but I had never seen it. And all these other strange skin infections began showing up because their immune systems were nonexistent. I'll always remember not knowing what was going on."[187]

But what also occupied him in the early 1980s was a chance to get more involved in treating a disease that had fascinated him since his residency days at Atlanta's Grady Memorial Hospital—Hansen's disease, or as it is better known, leprosy.

"Leprosy to me is an incredible and fascinating disease," he said. "It involves immunology, infectious diseases, and dermatology. It has a complete spectrum of activity. So many physicians have never seen or understand the disease."

Long before HIV became a stigmatized diagnosis, people with leprosy were feared and shunned. The disease was often seen as a curse or a punishment. It could destroy sight, disfigure the face, and damage the skin and nerves, leaving patients numb and susceptible to injury. Gangrenous fingers and toes often had to be amputated. In 1873, physician Gerhard Armauer Hansen in Bergen, Norway, discovered the rod-shaped bacterium that causes leprosy. But with no treatment until nearly 80 years later, fear of contagion led authorities to quarantine those displaying the disease's debilitating symptoms in so-called leper colonies.

A colony established in 1894 by the Daughters of Charity in Carville, Louisiana, later evolved into the National Hansen's Disease Center, operated by the US Public Health Service. Sulfone drugs to treat leprosy were developed there in the 1940s and the 1950s, although resistance to those drugs soon followed. The multidrug therapy used today was developed there in the 1970s.

Along with King Holmes—who years earlier had trained in epidemiology with University of Hawaii leprosy expert Robert Worth—Harnisch got to know researchers at the Carville center in the 1970s and to serve on its board. With his interest in leprosy and his training in both infectious diseases and dermatology, he became the informal go-to person in Washington and surrounding states for people seeking treatment. At that time, most of them were Vietnamese immigrants.

Then the Reagan administration began its drive to decentralize federal services and wind down Public Health Service hospitals, of which the Carville center was a part. In 1981, Harnisch got a phone call: would he be interested in opening an actual Hansen's disease clinic in Seattle, one of 12 initial sites throughout the country to receive federal funding?

"We knew we no longer had to institutionalize these people, but not that many physicians were familiar with treatment of the disease," Harnisch said. "I said fine." He received funding for himself, a nurse, and an administrative assistant.

The clinic first opened in the old Public Health Service Hospital, now the PacMed building, but like the Carville center, it, too, had begun winding down. When Holmes became chair of medicine at Harborview, the clinic moved there.

"The word leprosy still scares people," Harnisch said. "It's extraordinarily stigmatized. I had difficulty even getting a nurse to work for me or for other staff to work in the area where the clinic was."

Treatment renders patients noncontagious, and scientists have also learned that 95 percent of the world's population is not susceptible to infection with *Mycobacterium leprae*. For those who are susceptible, the rod-shaped bacterium is transmitted through close contact over time, often facilitated by poverty, poor nutrition, and crowding.

Yet the stigma remains. For that reason, the clinic bore no sign. Patients—sometimes afraid to even tell their families—were able to slip in and out without being noticed. The multidrug regimen must be continued over several years and getting patients to return required earning their trust. Like his counterparts treating HIV, Harnisch would often gently touch his patients' faces and hands, his way of showing that he did not fear them.

According to the CDC, between 200 and 250 new cases of leprosy are reported in the United States each year. The Harborview clinic, which is open one morning every other week, averages about six to eight new patients a year, in addition to established patients undergoing multiyear therapy. Today, they typically are immigrants from Mexico, the Philippines, India, Brazil, the Marshall Islands, and other Pacific islands.

Harnisch has continued to treat patients in the clinic for a half century as well as publishing research conducted there and with leprosy patients in Manaus, Brazil. Along the way, he trained other young physician-researchers interested in both dermatology and infectious diseases, including Philip Kirby, one of Bill Kirby's three children, all of whom trained as physicians. "They all inherited their father's soft, gentle personality," Harnisch said.

From infectious diseases to global health

AIDS was not Judith Wasserheit's focus when she began her training in infectious diseases in 1982, joining the same UW class of fellows as Ann Collier. What drew her to Seattle was a desire to learn clinical epidemiology.

"There was this guy here who was supposed to be one of the most incredible mentors in clinical epidemiological research," she said. "His name was King Holmes."[188]

Wasserheit knew the value of good mentors. Her first was her mother. The chair of special anatomy at the first podiatric medical school in the United States, her mother gave Wasserheit an unusual 13th birthday present: a cadaver. Mother and daughter spent their weekends at the morgue, dissecting the cadaver together.

Her family also bequeathed Wasserheit a love of travel, especially to less-trodden places. So after entering Harvard Medical School at age 19, she leapt at the chance to spend two months in Colombia providing primary care at a jungle hospital. After internships in internal medicine and in surgery at Columbia Presbyterian Medical Center, she did a senior residency in internal medicine at Emory University that included two months working in Khao-I-Dang, the largest Khmer refugee camp on the Thai-Cambodian border.

Those early experiences fueled a passion in what was not yet known as global health. The mentor she sought out would help create and define this new field, as would she.

Originally drawn to surgery because she liked being able to fix things, Wasserheit came to see infectious diseases in a similar way but on a larger scale and with the potential to have a greater impact on the health and human needs of lower-income countries. The subspecialty met her three career goals: to make a difference, to keep learning, and to have fun.

"The infectious disease field is, intellectually, just incredibly exciting," she said. "It touches on all the other subspecialties. There is always something to learn. And I like the people in ID. They went into medicine for the right reasons. And they tend to be people who are always up for adventure."

What's more, she added, "There is only one subspecialty where you can ask people where they traveled to, what pets they have, and who they're sleeping with, and that's infectious diseases. What more could you ask for, right?"

Admittedly, STIs were not, originally, at the top of her list of interests. She was drawn to Holmes for his epidemiological and mentoring skills rather than his research focus.

"I told him, 'If you work on STDs, I'll work on STDs. But that's not the reason I'm here,'" she said. "I guess he made his peace with that."

As her career would attest, she made her peace with his specialization as well, going on to become a leader in STD and HIV research and prevention herself.

"King basically created the field of academic STD research and education," she said. "By the time I got here in 1982, he was well on the way to making this a legitimate and respectable academic field."

When she arrived as a fellow, Holmes paired her with David Eschenbach, the ob-gyn who as one of Holmes's early fellows also trained in infectious diseases. Working with Holmes, Eschenbach, and Walt Stamm, Wasserheit was the lead author on a highly cited paper on the etiology of PID that clearly established *Chlamydia trachomatis* as an important causative organism.

Like all of Holmes's mentees, Wasserheit spent a fair amount of time waiting outside his office while other appointments ran over. Also like the others, she then had his full attention. Once, when she was getting ready to give her first presentation at an international meeting, she met with him at his house overlooking Lake Washington to practice beforehand.

She'd written out her talk. Holmes asked to see it. She handed the pages over and watched in shock as he tore them up.

"OK, Judy," he said. "Give me your talk."

"You might have wanted to strangle him," she said, with the equanimity that comes from the passage of decades. "But it was so wrapped up in the sense of 'I'm trying to help prepare you.' There was a tremendous sense of family and community here, in addition to the expertise and vision. Seattle was magical."

And it wasn't just Holmes. Also active in the training program were Stamm, Larry Corey, and Hunter Handsfield. Stamm and Corey shared their strengths in laboratory-based infectious-diseases research. Both had spent time at the CDC thinking about population-level impacts and epidemiology. Both were interested in the transition of laboratory-based interventions to large-scale, high-impact programs and policy. And while Wasserheit did not work directly with Handsfield, she admired—and later, emulated—his "Seattle model" for how universities and health departments could work together.

"They weren't at all limited by a narrow view of infectious diseases," said Wasserheit of her UW mentors. "They moved smoothly across those venues, dragging their mentees like me with them. They had a breadth of vision and they were really bright and really energetic and also warm and collegial. They were very into mentoring in the truest sense of the word—they adopted people for life."

In addition to her work with Eschenbach, Wasserheit found a way during her fellowship to reconnect with her earlier refugee research. She and clinical professor of medicine Elaine Jong cofounded the Southeast Asian Refugee Clinic at Harborview Medical Center to address the needs of Khmer and other camp refugees who had been relocated to Seattle. Now known as the International Medicine Clinic, it has expanded to see more than 10,000 patient visits a year by refugees and immigrants from around the world, including many from sub-Saharan Africa.

At her fellowship's end, Wasserheit went global with her research on the effects of STDs on maternal health. Working as a physician-scientist at the International Center for Diarrheal Disease Research in Bangladesh, she studied chlamydia, gonorrhea, trichomoniasis, HIV, and other reproductive-tract infections in a rural family planning clinic population, the first such population-based study in the Indian subcontinent.

In 1986, Ned Hook—who had been chief resident at Harborview when Wasserheit arrived at the UW and then a senior infectious-diseases fellow himself—recruited her to Johns Hopkins, where he had been recruited by former UW fellow Tom Quinn. Like Handsfield, who had been jointly appointed to head the Harborview STD clinic by the UW and Seattle–King County, Hook was an assistant professor of medicine as well as chief of Sexually Transmitted Disease Clinical Services at the Baltimore City Health Department. Wasserheit had a similar joint appointment and served as Hook's assistant chief.

"Because the UW group had this precocious view of how bench-to-bedside-to-community ought to work, Seattle was at the forefront of developing models for how universities and health departments ought to work together," Wasserheit said. "It's a really important concept—that those pieces ought to shake hands so that the health department had access to the analytic capacity of the university and the university had access to the data that the health department was accruing. That model came out of Seattle and then went to Baltimore and Birmingham and San Francisco."

In 1989, at age 34, the mentee who had told King Holmes that she wasn't especially interested in STIs moved to NIAID as the first chief of its newly established STD branch.

She found NIAID to be fairly conservative in that its research focused strictly on the biomedical, from pathogenesis to testing to the evaluation of drugs. She told her new boss, Anthony Fauci, that while she intended to establish a rigorous biomedical research program for STIs, she would also bring in behavioral science and what was then called operations research, now known as implementation science— studying methods and strategies to put proven health interventions into practice. Fauci was supportive, and hers became the first NIH branch to take such a big-picture approach.

"That broader orientation really came from my training with King. And Larry and Hunter and Walt were all very much part of that broader view of things," she said. "There was real vision here of how to connect the dots to make constructive change, as well as the training and the technical and interpersonal skills that are needed to be successful."

Three years later, she was recruited to lead the CDC's Division of STD/HIV Prevention, a position she held for a decade. There, she developed a training program for infectious-diseases fellows across the country so that these future ID researchers and clinicians could get experience working with CDC researchers and gain a public health perspective.

It was Larry Corey who brought Wasserheit back to Seattle in 2001 to be executive director of his new venture: the HIV Vaccine Trials Network. From that global endeavor, she moved five years later to become cochair of the UW's newly created Department of Global Health. In 2014, she succeeded its founding chair, her old mentor, King Holmes.

"The best people from around the country"

It was Seymour Klebanoff who drew Wes Van Voorhis to the University of Washington as an infectious-diseases fellow in 1986. A few years earlier, Klebanoff had gone back to Rockefeller University for a sabbatical. There he met Van Voorhis, who was working on a doctorate while also studying medicine at Cornell Medical College. Klebanoff impressed Van Voorhis as being both a great scientist and a genuinely nice person.

Van Voorhis no doubt impressed Klebanoff as well. He trained at Rockefeller with immunologists and cell biologists Zanvil A. Cohn and Ralph M. Steinman, who discovered a new class of cells called dendritic cells that are powerful initiators of immunity. (Steinman would share the 2011 Nobel Prize in Medicine for the discovery.) As Steinman's graduate student, Van Voorhis was the first to isolate dendritic cells from human blood.

"My mentor had done the work on mice, and my job was to find if humans had these cells," Van Voorhis said. "They did—and they were amazing. They orchestrated the whole immune response."[189]

After completing both his PhD and his medical degree in 1984, Van Voorhis did a short-track, two-year residency at the University of California, San Francisco. Knowing that he wanted to continue in infectious diseases, he applied to and was invited for interviews at nine fellowship programs around the country. By chance, he interviewed first at the University of Washington, arriving in Seattle after being awake on call all the night before. The infectious-diseases match process was not yet in place, so when, after a day of interviews, Klebanoff offered him the fellowship, Van Voorhis accepted on the spot.

It was not just the prospect of skipping eight additional sleep-deprived interviews that appealed to him.

"It was a really dynamic place that valued clinical care as well as research," he said. "I knew the University of Washington was one of the top four or five fellowship programs in the world, and I knew I loved Seymour. That's how I came to be here."

While at Rockefeller, Van Voorhis had spent a few months in Brazil working on leprosy and had become interested in the molecular biology of parasites. In Seattle, he worked with Harvey Eisen of Fred

Hutch on the intracellular parasite *Trypanosoma cruzi*, which causes Chagas disease, and, more generally, on the role of infectious agents in autoimmune diseases.

His clinical work, given the times, revolved around HIV/AIDS. Antiretroviral drugs were not yet in use, so like every physician of that era, he would care for patient after patient who would not survive the year.

As shattering as that was, he was buoyed by the division's all-hands-on-deck response to the crisis.

"Here's this huge problem, AIDS, that's killing a huge number of patients," he said. "People retooled themselves from other interests to work on AIDS. Our group swelled to dozens who worked on AIDS. That's been repeated as a new challenge comes up."

Klebanoff remained Van Voorhis's main career mentor, but Marvin Turck, King Holmes, and Hunter Handsfield—who oversaw the STD and, at the time, the HIV/AIDS clinics—were also key. He even had a chance to work clinically alongside Bill Kirby, whom he respected tremendously.

After his residency in San Francisco, Van Voorhis was particularly impressed by Harborview, which Marvin Turck ran from 1982 to 1988 as medical director.

"San Francisco General's hospital is under-resourced. It has fabulous UCSF attendings, but everything else is a total wreck," Van Voorhis said. "I came to Harborview and said, 'Holy cow—it really functions.' It has great resources. It has great nurses. I came to realize it was Marv's leadership. It was Marv working behind the scenes, making sure politically that bonds were passed. He had the gift of political savvy to make Harborview become the great place that it is."

In 1989, Turck became editor of *The Journal of Infectious Diseases*, the major academic journal for the field. He recruited a group from the UW to be associate editors, including King Holmes, Walt Stamm, Larry Corey, pediatrician and immunologist Chris Wilson, and molecular biologist Denise Galloway, whose research on human papillomavirus paved the way for the first HPV vaccine. Van Voorhis considered them to be "the gods of infectious diseases." When an associate editor with expertise in parasitology retired, Turck offered the role to Van Voorhis.

"I felt that really changed my career," he said. "Suddenly I knew most of the people in the country who were doing parasitology because they would send me their papers. It helped me understand how papers were written and what editors were looking for. Marv did that for so many people. It was a wonderful type of mentorship."

Van Voorhis was charmed by Turck's humor—and learned to accept his propensity to finish everyone's sentences. "He would come to a conclusion very quickly, which initially bothered everybody," he recalled, "but then you realized he was right 99.9 percent of the time. And you'd go, 'Holy cow, how did he do that?'"

Van Voorhis in turn teased Turck back, referred to the famous system for testing for antibiotic susceptibility that Turck contributed to as the "Kirby-Bauer-Turck" test most of the time but as the "Kirby-Bauer" test when he wanted to get Turck's ire up. It was a running joke between them.

When Walt Stamm succeeded Klebanoff as head of the infectious-diseases division in 1994, Stamm asked Van Voorhis to become the division's first fellowship program director rather than overseeing it himself. Given how rapidly the division itself was then growing, it made sense to separate the two jobs.

It used to be relatively unusual for fellows to stay on in Seattle. That changed late in Klebanoff's tenure as division head and under Stamm. Fellows who were able to get grant funding on interesting projects could stay on. And almost all of the growth occurred from within because the fellowship program provided such a strong pool of potential recruitees.

"The best people from around the country applied for the program," said Van Voorhis. "We were fortunate to be held in high regard. This continues to be the case. We had a wonderful pool to choose from, and then we were very thoughtful about who was chosen."

Van Voorhis was one of those top recruits who stayed on, succeeding Stamm in 2007 to lead the ID division for a decade.

The veterans

Before retiring in 1986, John Sherris wrote a leading textbook, *Sherris' Medical Microbiology: An Introduction to Microbiology*, with his wife Elizabeth doing the typing and indexing; first published in 1984, it is now in its sixth edition.

Marvin Turck spent much of the 1980s as an associate dean of the medical school and as medical director for Harborview Medical Center, where his political savvy contributed to the passage of three key bond proposals.

Seymour Klebanoff received a NIH MERIT Award in 1988 along with a string of other honors, including the Alexander Fleming (previously Bristol) Award of the Infectious Disease Society of America in 1993 and the Bristol-Myers Squibb Award for Distinguished Achievement in Infectious Disease Research in 1995. He stepped down from leading the division but still received a major grant at age 76.

Walt Stamm continued his research in UTIs and chlamydia and rose in leadership, serving as chief of infectious diseases at Harborview and, in 1994, succeeding Klebanoff as director of the UW division.

That was around the time that Robert Petersdorf returned to Seattle after retiring as president of the Association of American Medical Colleges. He became a distinguished physician at the Seattle VA Medical Center—the same position he had used to lure his mentor, Paul Beeson, to Seattle years earlier—and a special advisor to the UW dean of medicine. He would find that much had changed in the infectious-diseases division since he left in 1979, and not just because of HIV/AIDS.

But a familiar face remained, at least for a few more years. Bill Kirby had been appointed professor emeritus in 1985, but he still rounded on the wards of the university hospital, attended conferences, and held his wildly popular "plate rounds" in the clinical microbiology laboratory. He was a beloved daily presence at the school right up until the day he died in 1997 at age 82.

9

Generations

of Builders

So much about the Division of Allergy and Infectious Diseases has changed in the last 50 years, from the tremendous growth of the division to the advent of genetic testing. But to many in Seattle's infectious-diseases community, one difference stands out. Said Sheila Lukehart, who arrived as a fellow in 1979, the year Petersdorf left: "The thing that's changed the most is all the women."[190]

Lukehart went from being the only woman on the University of Washington infectious-diseases faculty to welcoming "an amazing group of really strong, brilliant women," including Ann Collier, Joan Kreiss, and Judy Wasserheit, who arrived as ID fellows in the 1980s, and Anna Wald and Jeanne Marrazzo, who began fellowships in the early 1990s.

This group of women interacted less with the division's initial builders than their own mentors had, although Petersdorf, Kirby, and Klebanoff were still present and involved in research, clinical care, or teaching.

It was the next generation of division builders who trained the women who began fellowships in the 1980s and 1990s. Still all male, they fostered a welcoming atmosphere for women that was considered unusual for that time. Two of their trainees—Wald and Marrazzo— would go on to lead ID divisions themselves at the UW and at the University of Alabama, Birmingham, respectively.

Drawn to HIV

When Wald arrived at the UW, Ann Collier, and Sheila Lukehart were established researchers, and women were making up more of each fellowship class. The faculty members active in the division's training program, including King Holmes, Hunter Handsfield, Larry Corey, and Walt Stamm, were "very supportive of women," Wald said, and they—and the women they had already trained and hired—became part of the UW's appeal. In addition, she added, "Women were more easily drawn into HIV and sexually transmitted diseases because of the aspect of sexuality and stigma."[191]

The first generation of physician-researchers to take on HIV, whether at the UW or elsewhere, were already trained or training as infectious-diseases specialists when the epidemic hit. They were mostly male and straight and had to learn about and earn the trust of the mostly gay patients first affected by the virus.

Once the epidemic was underway, many women as well as gay men entered infectious diseases specifically to battle AIDS. Both women and gay men could identify with the "outsider" status of sexual minorities and drug users most affected by HIV, Wald said. Her experience as an immigrant heightened that identification.

She came to the United States from Poland with her family when she was 13; both of her parents were in academic medicine, and her father was offered a visiting professorship. He soon decided to return to Poland, then still behind the iron curtain. But Wald's mother, having gotten her children out, was not going back.

Wald's parents were Holocaust survivors. Janina Prot-Wald had been a member of the Polish resistance and a field medic during the 1944 Warsaw uprising. Now she began the process of becoming licensed as a physician in her new country, practicing primary care and neurology near Boston. Wald was left to navigate school on her own, which was fine with her. She finished two grades in her first year, learning English as she went and focusing on science, with its universal language of mathematics.

As an undergraduate at Wesleyan, Wald was drawn to anthropology and comparative religion. It was one of her religion professors who suggested that her interests aligned well with the kind of interactions found in clinical medicine.

Wald entered New York's Mount Sinai School of Medicine in 1981 intending to become a primary care physician. By the time she graduated, AIDS cases had exploded. When she started her residency in internal medicine at Boston City Hospital in 1985, she asked to be assigned to a primary care clinic treating AIDS patients—only to be told that residents were barred due to the risk of infection.

"So of course, I dug my heels in, and I ended up doing that clinic," Wald said. That determination steered her career toward infectious diseases.

There was no treatment for AIDS when she started working in the inner-city Boston clinic as a resident. Like all clinicians in those harrowing early years, she could do little but offer comfort care. The next year, she taught providers at neighborhood clinics how to do basic HIV-related care: testing for the virus, taking sexual and drug-use histories, implementing infection control.

Wald at first resisted moving to Seattle when her then-boyfriend, now husband, Joel Kaufman, got a fellowship in occupational and environmental medicine at the University of Washington. But he was persuasive, and so she looked for work. Her HIV experience landed her an interview with Larry Corey and Ann Collier and a job as a research clinician with the AIDS Clinical Trials Unit. There, she enrolled participants, oversaw their care, and learned how to conduct clinical trials.

When Corey's herpesvirus grant was renewed, he asked Wald to join the project. She did, and a decades-long collaboration commenced. Wald began a senior fellowship in infectious diseases in 1991 and focused on the epidemiology, natural history, and immunobiology of herpes simplex infection. In addition to the fellowship, she finished a master's degree in epidemiology in 1994.

"A leader with a voice and a heart"

Jeanne Marrazzo, who began her UW fellowship a year after Wald, in 1992, was drawn to infectious diseases by a desire to work in HIV, particularly HIV in women. Her role model was her mother, a nurse who, in the later stages of her career, took care of young gay men who had gone home to northeastern Pennsylvania to die with their families.

"It really emphasized the humanism that I think embodies the best parts of medicine," Marrazzo wrote. "There were people at that time who were refusing to take care of those patients, so my mom was really strong and uncompromising about the fact that caring for them was her job, and she was going to do it."[192]

Already enamored of biology—she'd originally considered becoming an ornithologist or a marine biologist—Marrazzo received her medical degree in 1988 from Jefferson Medical College in Philadelphia and did her internship and residency in internal medicine at Yale-New Haven Hospital. As had been Wald's experience in Boston a few years earlier, AIDS was rampaging through the community served by the hospital. And there was still no treatment.

It was during her residency that Marrazzo became focused on women's vulnerability to HIV and other infections. In addition to caring for many young men with AIDS, she saw a side of the epidemic that remains largely unrecognized in the United States even today but predominates in sub-Saharan Africa—young women, often African American, who had been infected by boyfriends or husbands and often did not seek care until late in the disease.

"AIDS was really crushing young African-American women," Marrazzo said. "Their disease course was relentless. Everyone's was, of course, but they seemed to have fewer resources and less attention."[193]

She chose the UW for infectious-diseases training because of its strong emphasis on translational research—only Johns Hopkins and University of California San Francisco offered comparable opportunities to do dry lab research in epidemiology, she said. She was also impressed by the sheer number of, at that point, midcareer but advancing women faculty. Lukehart was already well known for her work in syphilis, and there was a cohort of women working in HIV, including Collier and Kreiss, whom Marrazzo described as "a force of nature."

And then there were peer mentors, like Wald, who became "the most devoted friend and colleague anyone could ask for."[194]

Hunter Handsfield became Marrazzo's primary mentor. "He was always supportive," she said. "He would not hesitate to pick up the phone on my behalf. He also connected me nationally to a lot of reproductive health people and opened up networks that have gone on for decades."[195]

Although Marrazzo worked with King Holmes only peripherally, she credits him with fostering an environment that supported women, citing Kreiss and HIV-prevention researcher Connie Celum, who had been a senior ID fellow under Holmes from 1989 to 1991.

"King really made their careers possible, bringing them up to the level of their potential," she said. "Larry did the same for Anna. I always got the sense that, if you did well, you were not limited by your gender, which I think was pretty unusual for that time."[196]

Celum, then a junior faculty member and the medical director of the STD clinic, also provided mentoring. She would go on to lead landmark studies contributing to the approval of PrEP, or Pre-Exposure Prophylaxis, to prevent HIV. Marrazzo also worked with Walt Stamm in his chlamydia lab at Harborview.

The UW infectious-diseases division, Marrazzo said, was filled with ambitious people who went for big grants.

"Seattle is just a draw for talent," she said. "The ID we learned there was just amazing, unparalleled. And the connections—everybody knew everybody in ID in Seattle."[197]

Like Wald, Marrazzo received a master in epidemiology in 1994, while also doing her fellowship. The following year she went to Atlanta for the STD/HIV Prevention Epidemiology and Public Health Fellowship begun by Judy Wasserheit.

"Vaginal health? Female-controlled prevention methods? These were not sexy concepts that attracted big names during my … training and early research career," she later wrote. "Luckily, through persistence and commitment and probably some measure of stubborn cluelessness, I connected with some brave visionary mentors who believed there was a future in this arena and who themselves had battled for sexual and reproductive health—women, LGBT people, others not always at the proverbial table when funding or policy priorities are set."[198]

Marrazzo joined the UW faculty in 1996, where she spent the next 21 years. She created a body of research that was truly interdisciplinary. She worked closely with David Fredricks to create a research program in the female vaginal microbiome that was ahead of its time. She ran a clinically based research program focused on vaginal health and vaginosis, did research in STDs in people infected with HIV, and studied the management of antibiotic resistance in gonorrhea.

She was particularly proud of her work as medical director of the Seattle STD/HIV Prevention and Training Center, which had been started by Stamm in 1979, then run by Celum for two years until Celum switched her focus to sub-Saharan Africa. The center trained providers in Washington, Oregon, Idaho, and Alaska.

Marrazzo was also codirector under Lukehart of the STD/AIDS Research Training Fellowship Program, which Lukehart had taken over from Holmes. "Working with her was an incredible course on putting a training grant together and teaching people to be researchers," Marrazzo said.[199]

She also served as president of the American STD Association and the International Society for STD Research and as associate editor of the journal *Sexually Transmitted Diseases.*

Described as "a leader with a voice and a heart,"[200] Marrazzo was recruited in 2016 to the University of Alabama Birmingham to succeed Ned Hook as director of its division of infectious diseases.

"A major thing that was unique about the University of Washington that very few institutions do is collaborative research. I'm trying to do that here," she said. "The other is mentoring and teaching. Now that I have this position of authority and power, I can put people together in ways that are informed by my background."[201]

Listening to patients

When Wald began working with Corey on herpesvirus research, the acyclovir studies had already been done; she started in on early clinical trials for two new antiviral drugs, valacyclovir and famciclovir, that built off of acyclovir. Although Corey was the principal investigator, he pulled Wald into meetings with Burroughs Wellcome and involved her in study design. She got to know Trudy Elion and became especially close friends with Gray Davis, a Burroughs-Wellcome clinical research scientist who was instrumental in developing acyclovir.

As Corey became more involved in HIV research, Wald in 1995 became director of the UW Virology Research Clinic at Harborview, which Corey had already made into a hub for herpes research. It is still one of the only clinics in the country focused predominantly on herpes. (Another of Corey's trainees, Rhoda Ashley Morrow, ran the

UW Virology lab at Seattle Children's, where she developed the gold-standard test for HSV-2 infection, the Western blot, still available only at the UW.)

Lifelong and incurable, genital herpes is one of the most frequent STIs worldwide. Once a person is infected, HSV hides out in nerve cells and reactivates periodically, sometimes causing symptoms, sometimes not. Even when symptoms are nonexistent, mild, or suppressed by medication, infected people can still spread the disease to their sexual partners, making a genital herpes diagnosis a source of embarrassment, shame, or stress that can interfere with relationships.

As her religion professor had predicted, Wald became known as an empathetic and supportive clinician, often answering emails late into the night and establishing long-term relationships with those suffering from this stigmatized infection. She recalled enrolling people with HIV into a study on genital herpes and finding that potential participants were far more concerned with the disclosure of herpes than AIDS.

"A patient is unlikely to remember who diagnosed them with strep throat, or a broken bone, but they will always remember the person who first told them that they have genital herpes," she wrote. "However, in issues relating to sexual health, many physicians are poorly trained and do not comprehend how important is their conduct, both verbal and nonverbal, on patients' adjustment to genital herpes."[202]

Wald's research contributions included showing that treatment by drugs in the acyclovir family can treat symptoms and—if taken daily—suppress outbreaks and reduce transmission, although only about 50 percent of the time. She showed that rapid viral expansion resulting in high viral loads can occur before a sore is visible or without symptoms at all, so that even people not experiencing obvious outbreaks can "shed" and transmit the virus to partners. She also helped determine that genital herpes increases the risk of acquiring HIV and is one of the main drivers of the HIV pandemic in sub-Saharan Africa.

In introducing Wald for the 2017 Distinguished Career Award from the American Sexually Transmitted Diseases Association, Corey credited her with contributing "paradigm-shifting clinical and translational research into the natural history of genital herpes."

In the award lecture, Wald said: "When I started my fellowship, my mentor Larry Corey guided me to listen to what the patients affected by the disease want—and they want to know about asymptomatic shedding and transmission. Since my original plan was to be a community-based primary care doctor, listening to patients seemed appropriate. And that, indeed, has been the focus of my career."[203]

Corey remained supportive of Wald's work on herpes but never shouldered in. The two did not always agree, but they enjoyed a free exchange of ideas—and a lot of "raucous laughter," Wald said. She has emulated this relationship in her own mentoring and also in her leadership of the infectious-diseases division, which she has directed since 2017.

"Sharing laughter," she said, "is very important."[204]

The optimist

Robert Petersdorf died in Seattle in 2006 at the age of 80, a month after his mentor, Paul Beeson, died in New Hampshire at the age of 97. But the generation of UW physician-researchers Petersdorf had mentored and influenced when he was chair of medicine continued to build.

One of the lessons Corey had learned from his own mentors, King Holmes and Marvin Turck, and from Petersdorf as well, was to let trainees pursue their own ideas and have their own sense of success. It was the culture of empowerment and autonomy so often expressed as "Off you go!"

He also learned from Holmes that there were no boundaries on what a physician-researcher could undertake. Holmes himself had gone from working on gonococcal diseases to creating the field of STD research to writing a textbook on STIs to focusing on the role of behavior in sexually transmitted infection control to, in 2006, founding the UW's Department of Global Health.

"King taught me you could re-create yourself," Corey said. "He was an incredible role model."[205]

A year after Joel Meyers died, Corey re-created himself. Having created a road map to drug development, he stepped away from the AIDS Clinical Trials Group, which he had led from 1987 to 1992, and shifted his focus from treatment research to finding a vaccine to prevent HIV.

He took a sabbatical in immunologist Ed Mocarski's lab at Stanford, returning to Seattle and retooling his laboratory with PhD-trained researchers who focused on immunology. He started a clinic for primary HIV infections, reinventing what he'd done with genital herpes. And he began his first scientific research with Anthony Fauci, the director of NIAID, whom he already knew well from the tumultuous years overseeing HIV treatment trials. Among the first papers they authored was one showing that latent pools of infected cells were established very early in the course of HIV infection, even if a patient gets started early on combination antiretroviral treatment within 10 days of acute infection.

When the UW lab at Children's Hospital got too cramped, he took the HIV part of his research back to the 11th floor of the PacMed building. He wrote his first HIV vaccine grant, working with a fellow from Australia, Stephen Kent, and bringing in UW immunologist Phil Greenberg.

In 1996, Corey was recruited to Fred Hutch to lead what is now the Vaccine and Infectious Disease Division. He had always worked closely with the Hutch when Meyers was alive, sharing resources and information between his virology lab and the infectious-diseases program that Meyers launched at the Hutch. Now Corey merged the two programs together in a more seamless way, with one virology laboratory that served them both.

"You weren't restricted," he said. "There was collaboration among the institutions based around people."

Even as he was building up the infectious-diseases division at the Hutch and embarking on new research in HIV and cancer, he undertook an additional venture. In 1998, NIAID's Anthony Fauci asked if Corey would develop and lead a second large network, this one to test HIV vaccines.

Then-Hutch president Lee Hartwell wanted to know whether Corey was sure such a venture would be successful.

"I said yeah, I think we should be able to do this in seven or eight years," Corey said. From the vantage point of two decades later, he acknowledged, "That was my innate optimism."[206]

He would need that optimism—and the confidence gained from his early success against herpes—to weather the disappointments to come. Finding a vaccine for HIV turned out to be a formidable scientific challenge.

"If I'd known how hard it was going to be—if [the setbacks] had come first—maybe I'd feel differently," he said, looking back. "But I'd had a lot of success and accolades, and it was sort of, 'OK, you can't walk away. If you're not willing to undertake a really tough challenge, who is?'"[207]

Corey assembled a team to run the HIV Vaccine Trials Network, or HVTN, which would be based at the Hutch. He also brought in Judith Wasserheit as HVTN executive director and Julie McElrath, who had done post-doctoral training in molecular immunology at Rockefeller University before working with Corey in the UW AIDS Clinical Trial Unit, to run the immunology lab. He lured George Counts back to Seattle to advise the network on recruiting and involving underserved populations.

Acting on one of the lessons he had taken from the bitter battles over AIDS treatments, one of Corey's earliest hires was Steve Wakefield, a longtime HIV and civil rights advocate, to do community outreach.

"Larry has a deep moral conviction to take care of the world that he's in with the talents that he has," Wakefield said. "Until he had grandchildren, I never remember him going on vacations. Now part of his drive to find a vaccine is so his grandchildren will never have to live with HIV."[208]

In addition to the scientific challenge, finding a vaccine for HIV also turned out to be a formidable structural challenge. Pharmaceutical companies, ordinarily involved in vaccine development and clinical trials, saw too much risk of failure and too little promise of market reward to take on HIV. So Corey and the team he assembled built first a national and then an international network, with clinical sites, researchers, outreach workers, and community advisors throughout the United States and in sub-Saharan Africa and South America. The sheer scale of the network made their work akin to running logistics operations for the Army or the Navy.

At the time, little vaccine research was done in the developing world, much less involving local researchers and communities. The HVTN developed standards for how to engage and collaborate with affected communities, how to address the public's fears about medical research, and how to expand training and mentoring to local collaborators.

Out of that research has come, if not yet a vaccine, new technologies for looking at immune responses and wide knowledge of the types of viral vectors that can be used to elicit different immune responses. These and other new concepts for approaching vaccine development have been put to use in developing vaccines for Ebola, tuberculosis, dengue, and cancers.

Even as Corey continued to work on finding an HIV vaccine, the network he put in place and the vaccine advances it discovered would come to play key roles in a future and even more urgent pandemic.

Wisdom and grace

While Corey was re-creating himself as a leader in vaccine development, Walt Stamm was leading the UW infectious-diseases division, succeeding Seymour Klebanoff as chair in 1994. Leadership came naturally to him, just as it had in high school, college, and throughout his career.

Early on, Stamm had risen to be chief of the hospital infections branch of the CDC's EIS. He returned to Seattle to be chief resident at Harborview and then chief of infectious diseases there. He oversaw the full ID division for 13 years, guiding its growth from 25 to 75 faculty, with a major expansion in federal research support.

"He had gravitas. He was charismatic," said Wes Van Voorhis. "When he walked into a room, the place lit up." Stamm and his wife, Peggy, were like "a happy Jack and Jackie Kennedy," Van Voorhis said.[209]

Stamm died in December 2009 from melanoma, about 15 months after Peggy died of ovarian cancer. He was 64. A decade later, his former colleagues and mentees can't talk about him without tearing up.

"I have never gotten over the grief of losing Walter," said one of his oldest friends, Lucy Tompkins.[210]

Both Stamm and Klebanoff before him were known for combining an intense focus on science with an easygoing personal style. Each was a good listener, but Stamm was by far the quieter of the two—so reserved, in fact, that others were sometimes mystified by all he could accomplish.

"He would seemingly not be doing much, and all of a sudden, all this incredible stuff gets done," said David Eschenbach. "It was his personality—he was very organized."[211]

Take his famously—some would say infamously—tidy desk.

Corey, who often said that his and Stamm's decades-long friendship made them an "academic odd couple," tells one of the best tidy-desk stories. As grant deadlines closed in, Corey's office would be "strewn with papers, cans of diet coke, and gum wrappers everywhere, a box of Cheerios for sustenance and brain food, the staff hysterical with activity, articles, drafts, writing implements on every surface, people running in and out of the office suite, voices on edge and at decibel levels." In other words, normal.

But in Stamm's office, everything was calm: no papers on the desk, no binders out of order. The only detectable sign of the season was the pencils—blunt instead of sharpened—but still precisely arranged on the desk. "It was as if some Danish modern designer was about to take a picture of the office," Corey said.[212]

And it wasn't just his desk.

Ann Collier remembered a time when UW Medicine sent someone to train everyone in the division on (insert eye roll here) "best practices" for documenting patient records. This was before electronic records, so all notes were handwritten. As an example of what *not* to do, the trainer held up a patient note without saying who had submitted it. But because Stamm's handwriting was as neat and elegant as everything else about him, everyone immediately recognized it as his.

Moreover, they all vehemently disagreed with the trainer's assessment.

"It had every relevant thing you need in an ID note—age, sex, where the person had traveled, what they had eaten, what they had been exposed to," Collier recalled. "It was perfect. And here is this woman saying, 'This is terrible. You can't bill, it doesn't have enough of x, it doesn't have enough of y, it doesn't have enough of z.' And we're all saying, 'This is garbage.'"[213]

It's telling that everyone has a story about a guy known for being quiet.

As an example of Stamm's unflappability, Judy Wasserheit recalled how one year, for his birthday, his executive assistant, Mary Fielder, arranged to have a kind of reverse-striptease during ID grand rounds. Yes, it was another era, but the notion was that, rather than performing a striptease herself, the stripper would strip *Stamm*.

"I'm a fellow, and I'm sitting in the front row next to Marvin Turck," who was then medical director of Harborview, Wasserheit said. "Walt starts presenting a case, and the birthday present walks in and starts to take off Walt's jacket, undo his tie, and then moves to unbuckle his belt. Marv is having a cat, sitting next to me. He's saying, 'Judy, what should I do? We can't have this at Harborview!'"[214]

But Stamm, being Stamm, handled it with his usual cool.

"He just scoops her under his arm, and says, 'I think it's time for us to leave,'" Wasserheit said. "It was hysterical. And it was vintage Walt."

Years later, when Wasserheit was working for the federal government and feeling a bit overwhelmed, she encountered Stamm at a meeting and asked if he ever felt that way.

"And he said to me, 'You know, Judy, I actually do. I go through these phases when I get totally overcommitted, and then I just have to go back and stop committing to things or wrap things up. Actually, it's really hard.'"

That admission—from always-organized Walt Stamm!—was comforting. "It was like, oh my God, even Walt Stamm gets overwhelmed," Wasserheit said. "We had this great talk about this, and he coached me on how to handle it."

That, too, was vintage Stamm: attentive, generous, instilling a "you can do this" confidence.

Stamm's research contributions were considerable. He maintained his focus on UTIs, chlamydia and other STIs, and hospital-acquired infections. He showed, for example, through a series of clinical trials that most UTIs and STIs could be cured with lower doses of antibiotics over shorter periods of time, minimizing the side effects of treatment and lessening the chances for resistance to develop.

He was best known for his work clarifying the role that chlamydia played in PID, a stealthy disease that often had no symptoms but could cause infertility or ectopic pregnancy. Testing for chlamydia involved time-consuming pelvic exams and laboratory tests, and since it could be asymptomatic, even knowing who to test was challenging. Stamm developed several rapid and sensitive tests and showed that screening women for chlamydia could sharply reduce the incidence of PID. Such screening programs were subsequently widely introduced in the United States and Europe—starting with Hunter Handsfield's Seattle–King County STD Clinic—markedly reducing the frequency of PID and its effects.

"He was a powerful influence in American infectious disease circles and at the UW," said Handsfield.[215]

Understated but nurturing, Stamm was adored by his trainees, said Sheila Lukehart. As division chair, he supported women's careers and, like the best managers (or parents), shielded the faculty from larger university worries. Memorable Christmas parties were held at the café Peggy Stamm co-owned in Madison Park.

Tom Quinn credits Stamm with teaching him how to balance academia and family.

"He was devoted to his family, and he was an avid skier, an avid golfer, and an avid tennis player," Quinn said. "He would do them with his wife and kids. He could do that because of how organized he was. When you're not in total disarray, you can spend time with your family."[216]

Stamm played other key leadership roles. He was one of the founders of the Urinary Tract Infection Commission, a global collaborative effort to promote excellence in UTI research. He was active in the Infectious Disease Society of America, serving as president in 2005. The premier association for ID researchers and clinicians, it was a descendent, of sorts, of Paul Beeson and Robert Petersdorf's beloved "Pus Club."

Like Petersdorf—except without the gruffness—Stamm would listen attentively to a contentious faculty or committee discussion and find the thread of consensus that allowed sparring parties to nod and move on.

Both Walt and Peggy Stamm described the year 2000 as their favorite year. On sabbatical in Geneva, Stamm worked for WHO. The family skied the Alps.

That was also the year and place that Peggy Stamm was diagnosed with cancer. She battled it for eight years, always willing to try new treatments.

When Stamm stepped down in the last year to care for her, Wes Van Voorhis became division head—though not without trepidation.

"You want to take over from an awful leader and transform something, not from a beloved leader who's doing a great job," Van Voorhis said. "My deepest fear was that people would say—what's that famous quote?—'You're no Jack Kennedy.'"

Van Voorhis asked Stamm for advice, noting how different they were. The words "quiet" and "unflappable" may have been mentioned, along with "I'm not that way."

Here is where Stamm's dry wit came in.

"I said, 'Walt, you've done such a great job with this division, I'm a little frightened stepping into your shoes,'" Van Voorhis recalled. "He said, 'Maybe just don't say so much.'"

As Peggy's treatment options dwindled, Corey, always close, became Stamm's confidant and sounding board. Then, four months after her death in July 2008, came Stamm's own diagnosis of metastatic melanoma, with lesions in his lung, liver, and brain. Corey became his friend's medical liaison and advocate, consulting with experts at Fred Hutch and around the world, including researchers at the NIH who were working on treatments that would soon lift the death sentence for some stage 4 melanoma patients.

"Larry took such care of Walt at the end," said Wasserheit.

But like Corey's beloved brother-in-law, who died of a now-treatable fungal infection, Stamm died before the new treatments that may have saved him were ready.

NIAID's Anthony Fauci remembered Stamm as one of the giants of infectious diseases and cited his work in the diagnosis and treatment of genitourinary infections, particularly those that result in PID, causing infertility.

"There are a lot of happy mothers out there now because of the work of Walt Stamm," Fauci said.[217]

In eulogizing his friend of almost 30 years, Corey told stories—about the infamously neat desk, about the calm consensus-building in faculty meetings, about the dignity that lasted through the end. He called on everyone present to remember Stamm and "the wisdom and grace with which he lived."[218]

Clearly, they have done so.

10

Postscript:

COVID-19

HIV had served as a warning that new and deadly pathogens could and would emerge. And emerge they did. In 2003, a novel coronavirus named SARS-CoV killed more than 700 people in 26 countries before being contained after about four months. A second novel coronavirus, MERS-CoV, emerged in the Middle East in 2012 and has since killed more than 800 people, mostly in Saudi Arabia.[219]

The Ebola virus, which Peter Piot had helped identify in the Democratic Republic of Congo in 1976 and which reemerged periodically over the next decades, caused an outbreak across three West African countries in 2014–2016 that killed more than 11,000 people. The mosquito-borne Zika virus, a flavivirus first found to infect humans in Uganda and Tanzania in 1952, caused an epidemic in Brazil in 2015 that included a new and troubling complication—babies born with microcephaly.

And in 2020, the viral pandemic that microbiologist John Sherris had warned about decades earlier in his final lecture exploded across the world. It was not caused by an influenza virus like the 1918 flu that had been the subject of Sherris's 1986 retirement talk. The culprit was a novel coronavirus named SARS-CoV-2. And Seattle, for a time, became ground zero in the unfolding pandemic.

That its infectious-diseases community was ready is a testament to the founders and early builders who are the subject of this history.

Even more quickly than researchers had remade their labs when HIV/AIDS emerged in the 1980s, many pivoted to focus on the virus behind the still mystifying new illness. The urgency was warranted. SARS-CoV-2 spread globally at a speed Larry Corey called unprecedented.

"I've seen other pathogens in my life, and certainly HIV is a formidable pathogen," Corey said in May 2020. "But we're dealing with a pathogen that's infected over 4 million people in a five-month period. And we're still counting."[220]

By September 2021, the World Health Organization reported more than 232 million confirmed cases and more than 4.7 million deaths.[221]

"We never considered saying no"

Just as the UW's expertise in STDs developed under King Holmes and his early fellows set Seattle up to lead the battle against AIDS, the knowledge, tools, and techniques developed to fight HIV would in turn play a key role in responding to the new threat of SARS-CoV-2. Innovations in diagnostics and hard-won insights into immunology that took years or decades to figure out for HIV were repurposed for the novel coronavirus, saving critical time.

First reports of a mysterious pneumonia emerged from Wuhan, China, in the waning days of 2019. On January 10, 2020, Chinese scientists identified the pathogen behind the cluster of cases as a coronavirus and published an initial genome sequence.

Five days after that, a man who lived in the Seattle suburbs returned from visiting relatives in Wuhan and began to feel ill. He would become the first reported case in the United States of COVID-19, the disease caused by the new virus.

The Seattle man went to a local urgent care center with flu-like symptoms on January 19. He told the clinician on duty that he had been in Wuhan, and the clinician notified local and state health departments and the CDC, then sent swab and serum samples by overnight flight to the CDC for testing. The CDC, using a just-developed test, confirmed the diagnosis the following day and called Providence Regional Medical Center in Everett, just north of Seattle, to ask if it would admit the 35-year-old man.

"We never considered saying no," said George Diaz, a Providence in-hospital infectious-diseases specialist who had completed an ID fellowship at the University of Washington in 2005.[222]

Diaz had been preparing for such a moment since 2015, when Providence Regional had been designated to admit potential Ebola patients during the West Africa outbreak. The hospital was not needed in that instance, but it had designed space to be converted into physical isolation units, with negative air pressure and a robot equipped with a camera, microphone, and stethoscope that can be operated from an adjoining room. Diaz regularly drilled his team on protective gear and isolation protocols.

The patient was transported via a plastic-enclosed isolation gurney to Providence Regional late on January 20. He was admitted for observation with just a cough and no fever, but his condition deteriorated six days later into pneumonia. With no playbook for treating the new disease, Diaz, on the CDC's advice, tried intravenous remdesivir. The 11-year-old experimental drug had been developed to treat Ebola but had little success; it had, however, showed promise against SARS and MERS.

The patient recovered, and Diaz's paper on the compassionate use of remdesivir was published in the *New England Journal of Medicine* on March 5. Later studies, including some done by Seattle-area researchers, would show that patients who received remdesivir had a 31 percent faster time to recovery.

Diaz was not alone among Seattle infectious-diseases specialists to take on COVID-19.

Helen Chu, a UW assistant professor in the ID division, and Fred Hutch–based evolutionary and computational biologist Trevor Bedford first detected community spread of the novel coronavirus, prompting Washington state government officials and private companies to send workers home and begin locking down the community, saving lives.

The University of Washington Medical Center virology laboratory became one of the first clinical laboratories nationwide to offer testing for SARS-CoV-2, a contribution that proved critical given that the test kits first distributed by the CDC to state and county public laboratories contained a flawed reagent, setting testing back in the critical early weeks.

Other UW-trained ID experts, both veterans and rising stars, worked around the clock on COVID-19. Among them was Larry

Corey, who, at the NIH's request, harnessed the global HIV Vaccine Trials Network and partnered with two other clinical trial groups to assess promising vaccines and monoclonal antibodies.

"The only way out of the epidemic is through science," Corey said. "And I think we are going to see what the scientific community can do."[223]

The new epicenter: Seattle

Helen Chu had not particularly planned to study respiratory viruses when she chose the UW for her infectious-diseases fellowship in 2009. As a student at Duke University Medical School, she had spent a year in East Africa researching home-based HIV testing, and she wanted to continue to work in resource-poor communities. "I wanted to go to a program where the global health presence was strong enough that I could do a lot of work in another country," she said. "The UW was the only program in the U.S. that had that."[224]

But life intervened, and Chu arrived in Seattle with a newborn, which made working abroad for long periods tricky. Then, in the first year of her fellowship, she encountered H1N1, the first global flu pandemic virus in 40 years. She pivoted to flu and found a mentor in Seattle Children's virologist Janet Englund. From a second mentor, Jane Kuypers, director of UW's Molecular Virology Development Laboratory, Chu learned how to do PCR, write a protocol, and other bench-science basics.

As her children got older, Chu ventured abroad to do a clinical trial of a flu vaccine for pregnant women in Nepal, traveling on the back of a midwife-driven motorcycle. She also worked with a low-resource community closer by—Seattle's homeless population. By the time she finished her fellowship in 2012, she'd found a niche: respiratory viruses in otherwise healthy adults.

She was perfectly situated for COVID-19.

Chu by then was lead clinician for the Seattle Flu Study, an innovative—and, typical of Seattle, collaborative—effort launched in 2018 and involving the Brotman Baty Institute, which includes researchers from UW Medicine, Seattle Children's, and Fred Hutch. The Flu Study distributed and collected nasal-swab home test kits from Puget Sound residents with flu-like symptoms, with the goal of developing strategies for detecting, monitoring, and controlling flu outbreaks.

Trevor Bedford, the Flu Study's Fred Hutch–based codirector, used genetic sequencing to track the spread. He also monitored flu internationally; previously, he had tracked the spread of Zika in South America and Ebola in West Africa.

Bedford turned his attention to the novel coronavirus as soon as Chinese scientists published its genome. In addition, Lea Starita, a research assistant professor at the UW Department of Genome Sciences and codirector of the Brotman Baty Advanced Technology Lab, promptly designed an assay to test for the new coronavirus.

Once the first patient was identified in Seattle on January 20, local health officials immediately began tracing his contacts. But Chu and her collaborators had another way to find out if the virus was spreading in the community: they could test the samples collected for the ongoing Flu Study.

"It seemed clear to me, as an epidemiologist and a clinician, that if we looked for it, we would probably find it," Chu said. "If we didn't find it, that would be a good thing—but we needed to look."[225]

The Flu Study tested for the presence of 27 respiratory pathogens, including influenza A/B, rhinovirus, enterovirus, adenovirus, and human coronaviruses known to cause colds. But the researchers' attempt to use their customized genetic test for SARS-CoV-2 ran into delays getting government approval both to repurpose the study and to use an unapproved test. After weeks of frustrating back and forth, Chu and her team decided to test for the novel coronavirus anyway; to not do so in a public emergency, they reasoned, would be unethical.

They began on February 25. Almost immediately, they found a local Washington teenager with no travel history who tested positive for the new virus. The researchers immediately notified public health officials, who were able to intercept the student five minutes after he'd returned to high school after staying home sick.

Chu recalled thinking, "It's just everywhere already."[226]

Chu's and Bedford's finding of community spread prompted government officials and private companies to take action. By the first week of March, many of the region's largest employers, including Microsoft and Amazon, sent employees home to work. Over the following weeks, Washington Governor Jay Inslee called for social distancing, closed down bars and restaurants, and limited the size of public gatherings. The University of Washington shifted to online classes.

Epidemiologist Eric Feigl-Ding of Harvard Chan School of Public Health called Chu "a true American hero" for her persistence in testing and for sounding an early warning. "Without her, the epidemic would have been 10 times worse," he said.[227]

Chu also was coinvestigator with ID division head Anna Wald—another of her mentors—of a multisite study of remdesivir. She worked with Fred Hutch collaborators on discovering monoclonal antibodies and looking for correlates of risk and of protection. She launched a study of COVID-19 in Seattle's homeless community and also began a study following COVID-19 survivors, including Seattle's first patient, over the long term.

"It's remarkable to me how much we've been at the forefront of this," she said, of Seattle-based infectious-diseases researchers' work on SARS-CoV-2. "At first, I thought it was because the virus came here first, so everyone had a head start. But I don't think that's the case. There's so much depth in the research infrastructure and talent. It does seem like we're making major contributions for every piece of it—the epidemiology, the diagnostics, the vaccine."[228]

"Repeat after me: emergency"

A key part of that infrastructure was the UW Medicine Virology Laboratory, whose origins go back to Corey's and Joel Meyers's early days. Virologist Keith Jerome, the lab director, and immunologist/epidemiologist Alex Greninger, its codirector, began developing a polymerase chain reaction test for the novel coronavirus the day after Chinese scientists published the virus's genome in January. But, like Chu and her team, they ran into roadblocks getting approval to use the test.

On January 31, Health and Human Services Secretary Alex Azar declared a public health emergency, which, counterintuitively, triggered tighter restrictions on tests developed by academic labs. Typically, such labs can make and use their own tests without government approval as long as the tests are not sold but used in their own facilities. Now the UW lab would have to get an Emergency Use Authorization from the Food and Drug Administration, which required tortuous paperwork. Greninger spent 100 hours filling out forms, only to be told the FDA would not accept them because he had emailed them rather than burning copies onto a disk and mailing the hard disk to the Document Control Center in suburban Washington, D.C.

"Repeat after me, emergency," Greninger emailed a colleague in exasperation.[229]

Finding positive-control material for validation was another roadblock, given that there were fewer than 14 confirmed COVID-19 cases in the country in mid-February. Obtaining what was available required both aggressive tracking and deft handling of the university's internal protocols.

At the same time, Greninger was making 70 phone calls a day to garner signatures from lab directors around the country, lobbying to speed up approval of academic laboratory–developed tests. On February 29, the FDA announced that it would allow certain academic labs, including the one at UW, to test people for the disease. The decision led to a blur of final validation studies and preparation of test guides and documentation.

Except for a quick break by Greninger to move his mother from her assisted-living facility to his apartment (long-term care and nursing facilities were being hit hard by the virus), the scientists and their team worked nonstop, seven days a week. Once testing began and volume increased, the lab became a 24-7 operation. With financial support from the UW, it quadrupled its high-throughput molecular biology equipment, recalled retired staff members, and recruited new hires. By the end of March, the lab was running 7,000 tests a day, fueled by breakfasts, lunches, and dinners delivered by a community of grateful supporters throughout Seattle.

"In the month of March, we went from testing only at the CDC to testing at the public health laboratories to testing with laboratory-developed tests in high-complexity laboratories to using FDA-authorized high-throughput analyzers to using point of care tests," Greninger and Jerome wrote. "It has been awesome to be able to contribute to the control of this virus."[230]

Others contributed as well. Joshua T. Schiffer, an infectious-diseases specialist and modeler at Fred Hutch who was a UW senior infectious-diseases fellow from 2007 to 2010, used computer simulations of viral transmission to gain insights into superspreading events. When COVID-19 began ravaging senior living homes, Alison Roxby, an assistant professor in the ID division who was a cofellow of Schiffer's, switched from researching HIV in newborns and adolescents to helping colleagues in UW Medicine coordinate on-site testing. Her team showed that an outbreak in an assisted-living facility could be prevented by testing all the staff and residents. In addition to her own studies, Wald, as head of the division, helped her colleagues overcome such hurdles as a lack of adequate personal protective equipment, a shortage of swabs, and the challenge of obtaining informed consent of study participants while practicing social distancing.

Wes Van Voorhis, former head of the ID division and now director of UW Medicine's Center for Emerging and Re-emerging Infectious Diseases, became one of a dozen investigators funded by NIAID to step up surveilling for spillover pathogens. Ann Collier led a research study on monoclonal antibodies as treatment for COVID-19. Former ID fellows Jeffrey Duchin (1995), Health Officer and chief of the Communicable Disease Epidemiology & Immunization Section for Public Health–Seattle & King County; John Lynch (2005), head of infection control at Harborview; and Steven Pergam (2005), head of infection control at the Seattle Cancer Care Alliance, became leading voices on COVID-19 prevention in Washington and around the country.

Said Larry Corey, "The Seattle science community is taking a rapid interest and pursuing a diversity of ideas, and it's terrific."[231]

The UW training—and influence—extended well beyond Washington state. Jeanne Marrazzo, head of the ID division at the University of Alabama, Birmingham, and a former UW faculty member and ID fellow, emerged as a leader not just in Alabama but nationwide.

And Peter Piot, who throughout his long career had survived close encounters with Ebola and other deadly diseases, had an all-too-personal confrontation with the coronavirus: he fell ill with COVID-19 in mid-March. The director of the London School of Hygiene & Tropical Medicine recovered after three long months, including a week in the hospital with severe pneumonia, isolated and fearing the worst.

"They got me, I sometimes thought," he said. "I have devoted my life to fighting viruses and finally, they get their revenge. For a week I balanced between heaven and Earth, on the edge of what could have been the end."[232]

Lessons from HIV

The novel coronavirus early on became Larry Corey's full-time obsession, seven days a week, with maybe five hours off to sleep. He immediately began working with his longtime HIV collaborators Anthony Fauci and John Mascola at NIAID and with NIH director Francis Collins on a plan to rapidly assess COVID-19 vaccines. In May 2020, the four published an article in *Science* outlining their approach.[233]

They urged an unprecedented public-private partnership among governments, academia, and philanthropies. Thinking ahead, not just about finding a vaccine that works but getting it manufactured and distributed into people's arms worldwide as rapidly as possible, they called for developing and licensing multiple vaccines using different platforms—proteins, viral vectors, and RNA and DNA technology. Having a range of vaccines would help protect varying populations—one might work better in older people, another in children or in pregnant women. And too, building on different platforms would spread the manufacturing burden, a significant barrier to overcome when the whole world needs vaccinating.

"No single production factory can make enough," said Corey. "Production is different for each [platform], so we will be able to use all vaccine production facilities because there are no overlaps."[234]

Using all production facilities would speed the manufacturing and distribution without compromising the safety of the clinical studies. And studies, too, could move quickly without taking shortcuts in the number of volunteers needed or endpoints required. How? Because of the existing HVTN's expertise and global reach. Principal investigators, clinicians, laboratory scientists, and statistical and computational modeling groups were already in place. Community education and outreach workers, schooled in HIV, knew how to reach the often-neglected populations disproportionately affected by both pandemics.

"We're standing on the 20-year infrastructure that we built," Corey said. "Thank goodness that exists. How else would we get 65 sites mobilized and ready to go in July, starting in March?"[235]

Pivoting was not the hard part.

"We are experienced at mobilizing clinical trials," he said. "What's different in this case, if you look at the speed and magnitude of what we want to achieve, is to be able to vaccinate the populace of not just the United States but the world. We're trying to vaccinate 7 billion people as fast as we can."[236]

By July, Corey had the COVID-19 Prevention Network, or CoVPN, up and running and was leading its operations center, based at Fred Hutch. One of the vaccines tested was an mRNA vaccine developed by NIAID's Vaccine Research Center and the drug company Moderna; in a large trial with 30,000 participants, it demonstrated 94 percent efficacy.

On December 18, 2020, the US Food and Drug Administration authorized the Moderna vaccine for emergency use.

Although the full history of the ongoing SARS-CoV-2 pandemic remains to be written, Seattle already has played a leading role. It built on the infrastructure created by Robert G. Petersdorf, William M.M. Kirby, John Sherris, Seymour Klebanoff, Marvin Turck, King Holmes—and so many others.

Afterword

Seymour Klebanoff died in 2016 at age 89. A tribute coauthored by Wes Van Voorhis named Klebanoff's scientific achievements and awards along with his "kindness, good humor, and incisive wit" and "enthusiasm and zest for investigation and discovery" that made him an inspiration and a sought-after mentor.[237]

Marvin Turck was named professor emeritus in 2017. At a party for his 50th anniversary at the UW, he received a chair inscribed on the back: "For insuring the future of the university." He was delighted with this acknowledgment that he had both trained generations of physicians and passed bonds to equip the hospital in which they practiced. When his memoirs were written, he said, he wanted to be remembered for his skills as a teacher and as a good politician.[238]

King Holmes became professor emeritus in 2020 after making the study of STIs part of the academic mainstream and the UW the center of such research—and later of HIV and global health research.

John Sherris retired in 1986 and lived long enough to see the global pandemic he warned about in his final lecture come to pass. He died peacefully at home in 2001 at age 100.

The infectious-diseases division that Robert G. Petersdorf, William M.M. Kirby, Sherris, Klebanoff, Turck, and Holmes launched in the 1950s and 1960s took form alongside the discipline's recognition as a distinct subspecialty. They and those they trained helped define the field.

Petersdorf's mentor, Paul Beeson, born in 1908, began his career when infectious diseases were such a common cause of illness and death that they were the domain of generalists, not specialists, with little but rudimentary treatments available besides comfort and support. Although individual physician-researchers such as Beeson at Yale and Maxwell Finland at Harvard had made names for themselves for researching infectious diseases and attracted young physician-scientists to train under them, it wasn't until antibiotics came into widespread use after World War II that ID divisions took off.

Some of them were started by Beeson's old friends in the Pus Club, like Barry Wood, who launched an ID division at Washington University in St. Louis in 1942. Theodore E. Woodward established one at the University of Maryland in 1948, where a few decades later, Turck's first fellow, Allan Ronald, did his initial training. Louis Weinstein ran the division at Boston University.

Among these early ID divisions was the one started at the UW in 1949 by Bill Kirby.

By the 1960s, formal infectious-diseases training programs and fellowships began to spring up across the country. Seattle's was one of the first and became one of the largest and most competitive.

The early builders' names live on in Seattle: the Paul B. Beeson Award honoring a faculty member exemplifying the scholarliness, humility, compassion, and integrity for which Beeson was known; the annual William M.M. Kirby dinner and lecture; the Marvin Turck Outstanding Teaching Award; the Joel Meyers Endowment Fellowship; the Walter E. Stamm Endowed Fellow Award; and the King K. Holmes Endowed Professorship in STDs and AIDS. Nationally, the Infectious Diseases Society of America memorialized its former president by establishing the Walter E. Stamm Mentor Award; among its recipients are Lucy Tompkins and George Counts, who felt especially honored because they so revered its namesake.

But more than in awards and fellowships, the early builders live on in the culture passed down by those who, after all, had always considered their biggest accomplishment to be training and mentoring. That culture, established by Petersdorf and Turck and continued by Holmes and Larry Corey, is one of empowerment and autonomy. It is also one of collaboration and camaraderie. And it is a culture that recognizes the connection between clinical practice and research.

The division was launched by leaders working in an era in which medicine was changing from being a healing art to a more science-based practice. But they never forgot the healing-art part of the equation. Later on, their trainees and their trainees' trainees extended the same care and attention they had learned to give patients to the communities involved in and affected by clinical trials.

The infectious-diseases field has changed dramatically since the days of Kirby and Petersdorf. Polymerase chain reaction–based tests can define a specific pathogen with unheard of speed and precision. Gene sequencing can detect transmission patterns and inform infection control practice. If Turck, Holmes, Stamm, and others recognized that disease syndromes such as PID could be caused by many different pathogens, Marrazzo's and others' work on the microbiome introduced the notion that a disease could be caused by communities of microbes rather than a single one. As UW respiratory virologist and 2009 ID fellow Helen Chu put it, "The ability to do science now requires so much expertise. It's much more group science, team science."

But then, team science is also part of the Seattle culture, at least since Holmes's time. It is culture as much as Seattle researchers' considerable accomplishments that make the UW infectious-diseases division so influential, long after its early leaders have gone.

Endnotes

Introduction

1   RG Petersdorf, "The Doctors' Dilemma" (*N Engl J Med*, 1978, 299, [PMID: 683236]), 628–34.

2   Author interview with Donald Kaye, Dec. 7, 2018.

3   Clement A. Finch, *Fulfilling the Dream: A History of the University of Washington School of Medicine, 1946 to 1988* (Medical Alumni Association, UW School of Medicine, 1990).

4   Marvin Turck, "Four Decades of Academia: A Personal Perspective" (*Infectious Diseases in Clinical Practice*, Nov. 2001), 411–414.

5   Author interview with Edward R. Hook III, Aug. 1, 2018.

6   The prevention agency's name has evolved over the years, from the Communicable Disease Center to the Center for Disease Control to, in 1992, the Centers for Disease Control and Prevention.

7   King K. Holmes, 1983; Paul J. Wiesner, 1989; Lawrence Corey, 1997; Peter Piot, 1998; Robert B. Jones, 1999; Walter E. Stamm, 2000; Robert C. Brunham, 2004; Sheila A. Lukehart, 2007; Edward W. Hook, 2008; Sharon Hillier, 2009; H. Hunter Handsfield, 2010; Thomas C. Quinn, 2011; David Martin, 2012; Anna Wald, 2015; Anne Marie Rompalo, 2016. Although not trained by King, UW professor and researcher E. Russell Alexander, the founding chair of UW's Department of Epidemiology and a mentor to many early ID

fellows, and Allan R. Ronald, Marv Turck's first fellow, also received achievement awards in 1984 and 1991, respectively.

8   Author interview with Ann Collier, Jan. 29, 2019.

9   Author interview with Jeanne Marrazzo, Feb. 15, 2019.

10   Author interview with Wes Van Voorhis, July 12, 2018.

11   Nancy F. Bauer, "Head of Hospital Resigns After 19 Months in Boston" (*The Harvard Crimson*, May 6, 1981).

12   Author interview with Ann Collier, Jan. 29, 2019.

Chapter 1: The Buillder

13   Robert G. Petersdorf, "The 1976 Paul B. Beeson Lecture: Some Observations on Experimental Endocarditis" (*The Yale Journal of Biology and Medicine*, 50, 1977).

14   Richard Rapport, *Physician: The Life of Paul Beeson* (Barricade Books Inc., 2001).

15   Robert G. Petersdorf, "Opening Remarks, Interplanetary Society Conference" (*The Journal of Infectious Diseases*, March 1999, 179, https://academic.oup.com/jid/article/179/Supplement_2/S289/2190704), S289–S290.

16   Richard Rapport, "Infectious Disease, Internal Medicine and Paul Beeson" (*Yale Medicine*, 2007-Winter).

17   Robert G. Petersdorf, "Opening Remarks" (Interplanetary Society Conference).

18   Ibid.

19   Robert G. Petersdorf, "Edward W. Hook, Jr.: A Tribute" (*The Journal of Infectious Diseases*, June 1999), 1217–1318.

20   Robert G. Petersdorf, "Opening Remarks" (Interplanetary Society Conference).

21   Ibid.

22   RG Petersdorf, PB Beeson, "Fever of Unexplained Origin: Report on 100 Cases" (*Medicine*, Baltimore, 1961, 40), 1–30.

23   Richard Root, Robert G. Petersdorf, "Dedication: to Paul Beeson, M.D." (*Journal of Infectious Diseases*, Vol. 179, Issue Supplement_2, March 1999), p. iv.

24   McDermott would go on to receive the Albert Lasker Award for his con-

tributions to the treatment and control of tuberculosis, with which he suffered. Wood, who trained at Hopkins, launched one of the country's first ID divisions at Washington University in St. Louis in 1942 when he was head of medicine there before returning to Hopkins as a vice president.

25   Robert G. Petersdorf, "Opening Remarks" (Interplanetary Society Conference).

26   Robert G. Petersdorf, "Tribute: William M.M. Kirby, M.D., 1914-1997" (*The Journal of Infectious Diseases*, 1998, 177), 1–2.

27   Author interview with Barbara Kirby, May 16, 2019.

28   William M.M. Kirby, "Properties of a Penicillin Inactivator Extracted from Penicillin-Resistant Staphylococci" (*The Journal of Clinical Investigation*, March 1945, 24[2]), 170–174.

29   Author interview with John Sherris, Nov. 10, 2017.

30   Ibid.

31   Ibid.

32   Clemson A. Finch, *Fulfilling the Dream: A History of the University of Washington School of Medicine, 1946-1988* (Medical Alumni Association, UW School of Medicine, 1990).

33   Personal correspondence from John Sherris to Barbara, Phillip, and Richard Kirby, Aug. 30, 2005.

Chapter 2: The Early Years

34   Clemson A. Finch, *Fulfilling the Dream: A History of the University of Washington School of Medicine, 1946-1988* (Medical Alumni Association, UW School of Medicine, 1990).

35   Author interview with Marvin Turck, Dec. 2016.

36   Marvin Turck, "Robert George Petersdorf" (Lives of the Fellows, Royal College of Physicians, http://munksroll.rcplondon.ac.uk/Biography/Details/5601).

37   Author interview with Marvin Turck, Dec. 2016.

38   Marvin Turck, "Four Decades of Academia: A Personal Perspective" (*Infectious Diseases in Clinical Practice*).

39   Ibid.

40   Marvin Turck, "Harry F. Dowling, M.D., 1904-2000" (The Journal of Infec-

tious Diseases, Vol. 185, Issue 8, April 15, 2002, https://doi.org/10.1086/339681), 1003–1004.

41   Author interview with Marvin Turck, Dec. 2016.

42   Marvin Turck, "Harry F. Dowling, M.D., 1904-2000" (The Journal of Infectious Diseases, Vol. 185, Issue 8, April 15, 2002, https://doi.org/10.1086/339681), 1003–1004.

43   Marvin Turck, "Four Decades of Academia: A Personal Perspective" (*Infectious Diseases in Clinical Practice*).

44   Ibid.

45   Ibid.

46   Author interview with George W. Counts, July 16, 2018.

47   Seymour J. Klebanoff, "Iodination of Bacteria: A Bactericidal Mechanism" (*Journal of Experimental Medicine*, Dec. 1967, 126 [6]), 1063–1078.

48   Henry Rosen, W. Conrad Liles, Wesley C. Van Voorhis, "Seymour J. Klebanoff: Discoverer of WBC Killing Mechanisms" (*PNAS*, 113 [46], Nov. 15, 2016, https://doi.org/10.1073/pnas.1616687113), 12891–12892.

49   Lawrence K. Altman, "Robert Petersdorf, 80, Major Force in U.S. Medicine, Dies" (*New York Times*, Oct. 6, 2006).

50   Author interview with Marvin Turck, Dec. 2016.

51   Gerard N. Burrow, *A History of Yale's School of Medicine* (Yale University Press, 2002).

52   Author interview with Marvin Turck, Dec. 2016.

53   Author interview with Barbara Kirby, May 16, 2019.

54   Author interview with John Sherris, Nov. 10, 2017.

55   Carole Beers, "Dr. Alfred Bauer, Foe of Diseases, Wars" (*Seattle Times*, Jan. 17, 1998).

56   William M.M. Kirby, "This Week's Citation Classic" (Institute for Scientific Information, Aug. 12, 1985, http://garfield.library.upenn.edu/classics1985/A1985ANC2900001.pdf).

57   Author interview with Barbara Kirby, May 16, 2019.

58   Author interview with Marvin Turck, Dec. 2016.

59   Ibid.

60   Ibid.

61   Author interview with Allan Ronald, Jan. 19, 2019.

62   Philip A. Mackowiak, "Theodore E. Woodward 1914-2005" (*Trans Am Clin Climatol Assoc.*, 117, 2006), lxviii-lxxi.

63 Larry Krotz, *Piecing the Puzzle: The Genesis of AIDS Research in Africa* (University of Manitoba Press, 1st ed., May 15, 2012).

64 Author interview with King Holmes, Aug. 18, 2018.

Chapter 3: Becoming a Force

65 Ibid.

66 Thomas H. Maugh II, "2 Years in a Closed Environment: 8 Pioneers Will Enter Their Own Little World" (*Los Angeles Times*, March 23, 1987).

67 Video: "King Holmes Profile in Leadership" (Everyday Leadership: Tools for Teaching Leadership and Management in Global Health, I-TECH, 2013).

68 Maj. Mark S. Rasnake, Maj. Nicholas G. Conger, Col. C. Kenneth McAllister, King K. Holmes, Col. Edmund C. Tramont, "History of U.S. Military Contributions to the Study of Sexually Transmitted Diseases" (*Military Medicine*, 170, 2005), 4–61.

69 Ibid.

70 Author interview with King Holmes, Aug. 18, 2018.

71 Ibid.

72 David A. Schwartz, *Medicine Science and Dreams: The Making of Physician-Scientists* e-book (Springer Science & Business Media, 2010).

73 Author interview with King Holmes, Aug. 18, 2018.

74 Video: "King Holmes Profile in Leadership" (Everyday Leadership: Tools for Teaching Leadership and Management in Global Health, I-TECH, 2013).

75 Author interview with King Holmes, March 22, 2019.

76 Author interview with King Holmes, April 19, 2018.

77 Author interview with King Holmes, Aug. 18, 2018.

78 U.S. House Committee on Interstate and Foreign Commerce Subcommittee on Public Health and Welfare, "Operation of Public Health Service Hospitals" (U.S. Government Printing Office, 1971).

79 Author interview with King Holmes, Aug. 18, 2019.

80 Ibid.

81 Author interview with King Holmes, March 22, 2019.

82 Rainer Storb, "Program Genealogies: Bone Marrow Transplantation at Fred Hutch" (*The Hematologist*, July-August 2016, Vol. 13, Issue 4).

83 Author interview with King Holmes, Nov. 16, 2017.

84 George W. Counts, "This Wondrous Adventure—The Journey of a Sharecropper's Son" (Courtesy of George W. Counts).

85 Barbara Berg, "A 'hard sell' for minority health" (Fred Hutchinson Cancer Research Center News, Nov. 7, 2002, https://www.fredhutch.org/en/news/center-news/2002/11/minority-health.html).

86 Author interview with George Counts, July 16, 2018.

87 Richard B. Guttler, Harry N. Beaty, "Minocycline in the Chemoprophylaxis of Meningococcal Disease" (*Antimicrobial Agents and Chemotherapy*, May 1972, https://aac.asm.org/content/aac/1/5/397.full.pdf), 397–402.

88 Author interview with George Counts, July 16, 2018.

89 Video: "King Holmes Profile in Leadership" (Everyday Leadership: Tools for Teaching Leadership and Management in Global Health, I-TECH, 2013).

90 Ibid.

Chapter 4: Shaping a New Field

91 PL Perine, HH Handsfield, KK Holmes, JH Blount, "Epidemiology of the Sexually Transmitted Diseases" (*Annual Review of Public Health*, Vol. 6:85-106, 1985).

92 Author interview with Hunter Handsfield, Feb. 5, 2018.

93 Ibid.

94 HH Handsfield, TO Lipman, JP Harnisch, E Tronca, KK Holmes, "Asymptomatic Gonorrhea in Men—Diagnosis, Natural Course, Prevalence and Significance" (*N Engl J Med*, 290[3], Jan. 17, 1974, doi: 10.1056/NEJM197401172900301, PMID: 4202519), 117–123.

95 Author interview with King Holmes, April 19, 2018.

96 Melissa K. Klein, "The Legacy of the 'Yellow Berets': The Vietnam War, the Doctor Draft, and the NIH Associate Training Program" manuscript (NIH History Office, National Institutes of Health, Bethesda, Maryland, 1998).

97 The Venereal Disease Division was later renamed the Division of STD Prevention.

98 Author interview with James Harnisch, March 22, 2019 (also source of subsequent quotes).

99   Author interview with King Holmes, April 19, 2018.

100   Author interview with David Eschenbach, Dec. 13, 2018 (also source of subsequent quotes unless noted).

101   D.A. Eschenbach, T.M. Buchanan, H.M. Pollock, P.S. Forsyth, E.R. Alexander, J.S. Lin, S.P. Wang, B.B. Wentworth, W.M. McCormack, K.K. Holmes, "Polymicrobial Etiology of Acute Pelvic Inflammatory Disease" (*N Engl J Med*, 293, 1975), 166–171.

102   American College of Physicians Laureate Award, US Navy Region (https://www.acponline.org/system/files/documents/about_acp/chapters/navy/laureate.pdf, Dec. 4, 1993).

103   The prevention agency's name has evolved over the years, from the Communicable Disease Center to the Center for Disease Control to, in 1992, the Centers for Disease Control and Prevention.

104   Author interview with King Holmes, April 19, 2018.

105   Robert G. Petersdorf, "The 1976 Paul B. Beeson Lecture: Some Observations on Experimental Endocarditis" (*The Yale Journal of Biology and Medicine*, 1977).

Chapter 5: Atlanta to Seattle

106   David Dale, "Walter E. Stamm, M.D., 1945-2009" (*Trans Am Clin Climatol Assoc.*, Vol. 122: 30, 2011).

107   Lawrence Corey, Steven E. Saltman, Michael F. Epstein, *Medicine in a Changing Society* (Saint Louis: The C.V. Mosby Company, 1972).

108   Author interview with Larry Corey, Aug. 21, 2018 (also source of subsequent quotes unless noted).

109   Larry Corey, Walt Stamm eulogy, 2009, courtesy of Larry Corey.

110   Ibid.

111   Mary Engel, "A Virus Researcher's 35 Years in the AIDS Trenches" (Fred Hutch News Service, June 13, 2016, https://www.fredhutch.org/en/news/center-news/2016/06/35-years-in-the-AIDS-trenches.html).

112   Rachel Tompa, "The miracle was you got to see some part of that person's life" (Fred Hutch News Service, June 7, 2016, https://www.fredhutch.org/en/news/center-news/2016/06/infectious-disease-pioneer-dr-joel-meyers-honored-inaugural-symposium.html).

113   Ibid.

114 Rachel Tompa, op. cit.

115 Stanley Falkow, "The Fortunate Professor" (*Annual Review of Microbiology*, 62:1, 2008), 1–18.

116 Larry Corey, "Raising the Consciousness for Identifying and Controlling Viral STDs: Fears and Frustrations" (Thomas Parran Award Lecture, Sexually Transmitted Diseases V. 25:2, February 1998).

117 Author interview with King Holmes, Aug. 8, 2018.

118 J. Leo, "The New Scarlet Letter: Herpes, an Incurable Virus, Threatens to Undo the Sexual Revolution" (*Time* magazine, 120(5), 1982).

119 Rainer Storb, "Program Genealogies: Bone Marrow Transplantation at Fred Hutch" (*The Hematologist*, Vol. 13, Issue 4, June 15, 2016).

120 Mary Engel, "'The successes kept you going': 40 Years of Bone Marrow Transplantation" (Fred Hutch News Service, March 27, 2015, https://www.fredhutch.org/en/news/center-news/2015/03/40-years-bone-marrow-transplantation.html).

121 Author interview with David Martin, Feb. 19, 2019 (also source of subsequent quotes unless otherwise noted).

122 Author interview with Lucy Tompkins, Feb. 15, 2019 (also source of subsequent quotes unless otherwise noted).

123 Walter Stamm, "Chlamydia Trachomatis—The Persistent Pathogen" (Thomas Parran Award Lecture, Sexually Transmitted Diseases, V. 28: 12, December 2001).

124 Rachel Tompa, op. cit.

125 Barbara Berg, "The Most Satisfying Thing I Do: Late Husband's Research Inspires Barbara Thrasher's Commitment to Fight Cancer" (*Quest* magazine, Fred Hutchinson Cancer Research Center, Spring 2003).

Chapter 6: STD Research Booms

126 Author interview with Sheila Lukehart, Dec. 5, 2018 (also source of subsequent quotes).

127 Author interview with Hunter Handsfield, Feb. 5, 2018.

128 Dan Vergano, "Sexual Diseases Research Award Renamed after Vote" (*USA TODAY*, April 11, 2013, https://www.usatoday.com/story/tech/sciencefair/2013/04/11/parran-award-renamed/2074771/).

129 Edward W. Hook III, Introduction to 2010 Parran Award.

130 Author interview with Marvin Turck, Dec. 2016.

131 Author interview with Edward W. Hook III, Aug. 8, 2018.

132 Marvin Turck, op. cit.

133 Edward W. Hook III interview, Aug. 8, 2018.

134 Edward W. Hook III interview, May 19, 2021.

135 Ibid.

136 Author interview with Robert Brunham, Feb. 18, 2019 (also source of subsequent quotes).

137 Cho-chou Kuo, "San-pin Wang, MD, MPH, DMSc 1920-2001" (*Sexually Transmitted Diseases*, Vol. 28:9, September 2001).

138 KK Holmes, HH Handsfield, SP Wang, BB Wentworth, M Turck, JB Anderson, ER Alexander, "Etiology of Nongonococcal Urethritis" (*N Engl J Med.*, 292[23], June 5, 1975), 1199–205.

139 Victoria A. Harden, "In Their Own Words… NIH Researchers Recall the Early Years of AIDS: Interview with Peter Piot" (NIH, Jan. 4, 2008).

140 Ibid.

141 Author interview with Peter Piot, Dec. 2, 2019.

142 Ibid.

143 Ibid.

144 Author interview with Thomas Quinn, Jan. 30, 2019 (also source of subsequent quotes unless noted).

145 Marvin Turck interview, op. cit.

146 Ronald Allan, introduction to 2004 Thomas Parran Award to Robert Brunham.

147 Thomas Quinn, op. cit.

Chapter 7: AIDS Changes Everything

148 Author interview with Larry Corey, Aug. 21, 2018.

149 Ibid.

150 Author interview with Hunter Handsfield, Feb. 5, 2018.

151 Ibid.

152 Author interview with Ann Collier, Jan. 29, 2019 (also source of subsequent quotes unless noted).

153   Hunter Handsfield interview by Lawrence Knopp (Seattle–King County Department of Public Health Oral History Project, Sept. 4, 2015, https://vimeo.com/147181093).

154   Author interview with Robert Wood, Aug. 10, 2021 (also source of other quotes unless otherwise noted).

155   Rosette Royale, "HIV/AIDS in Western Washington" (posted 9/28/2019 on HistoryLink.org https://www.historylink.org/File/20871).

156   Patricia McInturff interview by Lawrence Knopp (Seattle–King County Department of Public Health HIV-AIDS Oral History Project, Sept. 4, 2015, https://vimeo.com/146045620).

157   Robert Wood, Responding to AIDS: The Seattle–King County Department of Public Health, 1982–1996, interviewed August 2015.

158   Patricia McInturff, op. cit.

159   Responding to AIDS: The Seattle–King County Department of Public Health, 1982–1996 archives, https://kingcounty.gov/depts/records-licensing/archives/exhibits/RespondingtoAIDS/AIDS_Omnibus_Act.aspx.

160   Author interview with Larry Corey, Feb. 18, 2019.

161   Rita Rubin, "Collaboration and Conflict: Looking Back at the 30-Year History of the AIDS Clinical Trial Group" (*JAMA*, 314:24, Dec. 22/29, 2015, http://depts.washington.edu/actu/wordpress/wp-content/uploads/2016/01/Collaboration-and-Conflict-the-30-Year-History-of-the-ACTG.pdf).

162   Author interview with Larry Corey, Aug. 21, 2018.

163   Mary Engel, "A Virus Researcher's 35 Years in the AIDS Trenches" (Fred Hutch News Service, June 13, 2016, https://www.fredhutch.org/en/news/center-news/2016/06/35-years-in-the-AIDS-trenches.html).

164   Ibid.

165   EM Connor, RS Sperling, R Gelber, et al., "Reduction of Maternal-Infant Transmission of Human Immunodeficiency Virus Type 1 with Zidovudine Treatment: Pediatric AIDS Clinical Trials Group Protocol 076 Study Group" (*N Engl J Med*, 331, 1994), 1173–80.

166   Author interview with Allan Ronald, Jan. 19, 2019.

167   Sabrina Richards, "25 Powerful Years of HIV Research: Longstanding Mombasa Cohort Helps Answers Questions about HIV Risk and Transmission" (Fred Hutch News Service, Feb. 26, 2018).

168   John Maurice, "Peter Piot wins 2015 Canada Gairdner Global Health Award" (*The Lancet*, Vol. 385, Issue 9974, March 25, 2015, https://www.thelancet.com/journals/lancet/article/PIIS0140-6736(15)60610-9/fulltext).

169   Author interview with Peter Piot, Dec. 1, 2019.

170   Author interview with Larry Corey, Aug. 21, 2018.

171   Robert Wood interview, "Responding to AIDS: The Seattle–King County Department of Public Health 1982–1996" (The Legacy, LBGT Rights, 2016 (https://soundcloud.com/user-572142711/lgbt-rights).

172   Author interview with John Sherris, Nov. 10, 2017.

Chapter 8: A Diverse Portfolio of Research

173   Author interview with James Harnisch, March 22, 2019.

174   Barbara Berg, "An Early History of the Fred Hutchinson Cancer Research Center 1972 through 1981" (http://authors.fhcrc.org/624/1/FH-CRCHistoryProject.pdf, November 2003).

175   Rachel Tompa, "The miracle was you got to see some part of that person's life" (Fred Hutch News Service, June 7, 2016, https://www.fredhutch.org/en/news/center-news/2016/06/infectious-disease-pioneer-dr-joel-meyers-honored-inaugural-symposium.html).

176   E. Donnall Thomas, biographical statement, The Nobel Prize in Physiology or Medicine 1990, https://www.nobelprize.org/prizes/medicine/1990/thomas/facts/.

177   Mary Engel, "Inaugural Symposium Honors Dr. Joel Meyers" (Fred Hutch News Service, June 17, 2016, https://www.fredhutch.org/en/news/center-news/2016/06/aids-vaccine-hiv-infectious-disease-Immunocompromised.html).

178   Ibid.

179   Tompa, op. cit.

180   Engel, op. cit.

181   Author interview with Michael Boeckh, June 13, 2016.

182   Author interview with George Counts, July 16, 2018.

183   Engel, op. cit.

184   Author interview with George Counts, July 16, 2018 (also subsequent quotes unless noted).

185   GW Counts, "APIC and the 1985 position paper 'Listen to the Music'" (*American Journal of Infection Control*, 17[2], April 1989), 49–55.

186   V Berthaud, D Hewlett, "A Piece of History: The Legacy of George W. Counts and Underrepresented Populations" (*Journal of Infectious Diseases*,

222[Suppl 6], doi: 10.1093/infdis/jiaa215, PMID: 32926737, Sep. 14, 2020) S550–S553.

187   Author interview with Jim Harnisch, March 22, 2019.

188   Author interview with Judith Wasserheit, Jan. 1, 2019.

189   Author interview with Wes Van Voorhis, July 12, 2018.

Chapter 9: Generations of Builders

190   Author interview with Sheila Lukehart, Dec. 5, 2018.

191   Author interview with Anna Wald, Aug. 16, 2018.

192   Women in Medicine Spotlight: Jeanne Marrazzo, University of Arizona Birmingham Medicine, https://www.uabmedicine.org/diversity/-/asset_publisher/pK6OqSCC5sf8/content/women-in-medicine-spotlight-jeanne-marrazzo?inheritRedirect=false.

193   Author interview with Jeanne Marrazzo, Feb. 15, 2019.

194   Jeanne Marrazzo, American Sexually Transmitted Diseases Achievement Award acceptance speech, 2015, https://www.youtube.com/watch?v=MOUlFapcu4M&feature=youtu.be.

195   Author interview with Jeanne Marrazzo, Feb. 15, 2019.

196   Ibid.

197   Ibid.

198   "Hooked on ID With Jeanne Marrazzo" (*Infectious Disease News*, October 2019).

199   Author interview with Jeanne Marrazzo interview, Feb. 15, 2019.

200   J. Dennis Fortenberry, introduction to 2015 American Sexually Transmitted Diseases Association Achievement.

201   Author interview with Jeanne Marrazzo, Feb. 15, 2019.

202   Ibid.

203   Anna Wald, "Hermeneutics of Herpes: The American Sexually Transmitted Diseases Association Distinguished Career Award Lecture" (*Sexually Transmitted Diseases*, Vol. 4, Issue 1, January 2017), 2–6.

204   Author interview with Anna Wald, Aug. 16, 2018.

205   Author interview with Larry Corey, Aug. 21, 2018.

206   Larry Corey, Vaccine and Infectious Disease Division seminar, January 2016.

207 Mary Engel, "A Virus Researcher's 35 Years in the AIDS Trenches" (Fred Hutch News Service, June 13, 2016, https://www.fredhutch.org/en/news/center-news/2016/06/35-years-in-the-AIDS-trenches.html).

208 Ibid.

209 Author interview with Wes Van Voorhis, July 12, 2018 (also source of subsequent quotes).

210 Author interview with Lucy Tompkins, Feb. 15, 2019.

211 Author interview with David Eschenbach, Dec. 13, 2018.

212 Larry Corey, Walt Stamm eulogy, Dec. 2009.

213 Author interview with Ann Collier, Jan. 29, 2019.

214 Author interview with Judith Wasserheit, Jan. 1, 2019 (also source of subsequent quotes).

215 Author interview with Hunter Handsfield, Feb. 5, 2018.

216 Author interview with Thomas Quinn, Jan. 30, 2019.

217 Thomas H. Maugh II, "Walt Stamm Dies at 64" (*Los Angeles Times*, Dec. 26, 2009).

218 Larry Corey, Walt Stamm eulogy, December 2009.

Chapter 10: Postscript: COVID-19

219 "COVID-19, MERS & SARS" (National Institute of Allergy and Infectious Diseases, https://www.niaid.nih.gov/diseases-conditions/covid-19).

220 Luke Timmerman interview of Larry Corey, The Long Run podcast, May 13, 2020 (https://timmermanreport.com/2020/05/coronavirus-vaccine-strategy-larry-corey-on-the-long-run/).

221 WHO Coronavirus (COVID-19) Dashboard, Sept. 28, 2021.

222 Alice Park, "How Remdesivir Moved from Back Shelf to Best Hope for Treating COVID-19" (*Time* magazine, May 21, 2020).

223 Larry Corey interview with Tom Lynch, Fred Hutchinson Cancer Research Center webinar, June 5, 2020.

224 Author interview with Helen Chu, Aug. 27, 2020.

225 Ibid.

226 Sheri Fink and Mike Baker, "'It's Just Everywhere Already': How Delays in Testing Set Back the U.S. Coronavirus Response" (*New York Times*, March 10, 2020).

227 The Gee and Ursula Show, interview with Dr. Eric Feigl-Ding, KIRO Radio, March 11, 2020, https://omny.fm/shows/the-gee-and-ursula-show/harvard-epidemiologist-dr-eric-feigl-ding.

228 Author interview with Helen Chu, Aug. 27, 2020.

229 Shawn Boburg, Robert O'Harrow Jr., Neena Satija, Amy Goldstein, "Inside the Coronavirus Testing Failure: Alarm and Dismay among the Scientists Who Sought to Help" (*The Washington Post*, April 3, 2020, https://www.washingtonpost.com/investigations/2020/04/03/coronavirus-cdc-test-kits-public-health-labs/?arc404=true).

230 AL Greninger, KR Jerome, "The First Quarter of SARS-CoV-2 Testing: The University of Washington Medicine Experience" (*Journal of Clinical Microbiology*, Vol. 58, No. 8, July 2020, https://jcm.asm.org/content/58/8/e01416-20).

231 Sandi Doughton, "Drugs Touted by Trump, Blood from Recovered Patients: Seattle Scientists Seek Coronavirus Cures" (*Seattle Times*, March 30, 2020).

232 Dirk Draulans, "'Finally, a virus got me.' Scientist Who Fought Ebola and HIV Reflects on Facing Death from COVID-19" (*Science*, May 8, 2020, https://www.sciencemag.org/news/2020/05/finally-virus-got-me-scientist-who-fought-ebola-and-hiv-reflects-facing-death-covid-19).

233 L. Corey, J.R. Mascola, A.S. Fauci, F.S. Collins, "A Strategic Approach to COVID-19 Vaccine R&D" (*Science*, Vol. 368, Issue 6494, May 2020), 948–950.

234 Larry Corey interview with Tom Lynch, Fred Hutchinson Cancer Research Center webinar, June 5, 2020.

235 Ibid.

236 Ibid.

Afterword

237 Henry Rosen, W. Conrad Liles, Wesley C. Van Voorhis, "Seymour J. Klebanoff: Discoverer of WBC Killing Mechanisms" (*PNAS*, 113 [46], November 15, 2016, first published November 4, 2016, https://doi.org/10.1073/pnas.1616687113), 12891–12892.

238 Author interview with Marvin Turck, Dec. 2016.

Appendix

Key dates for ID research in Seattle

1946   UW School of Medicine founded.

1949   William M.M. Kirby recruited to head infectious diseases at UW.

1959   John Sherris recruited to head microbiology laboratory at newly opened UW Medical Center.

1960   Robert G. Petersdorf recruited to be chief of medicine at Harborview.

Marvin Turck assigned to Seattle by EIS and simultaneously becomes Petersdorf's first fellow.

E. Russell Alexander joins faculty; later, as chair of Department of Epidemiology, he will become an influential mentor for ID fellows.

1961   "Fever of Unexplained Origin," by Petersdorf and his Yale mentor, Paul Beeson, is published in *Medicine.*

George Kenny joins faculty; as chair of Department of Pathology, he will mentor ID fellows.

Harry Beaty trains as an ID fellow with Petersdorf.

1962   Seymour Klebanoff joins UW faculty.

1963   Infectious Diseases Society of America founded; Kirby is a charter member.

1964–
1979   Petersdorf is UW chair of medicine.

1964   Turck, after completing his residency, returns to UW as chief of infectious diseases at Harborview.

1965   Beaty joins faculty.

1965–
1968   Allan Ronald trains as Turck's first fellow, then trains in microbiology with Sherris.

1966   Kirby-Bauer-Sherris-Turck paper published in *American Journal of Clinical Pathology*.

1967   Klebanoff publishes landmark study on phagocytes in *Journal of Experimental Medicine*.

King K. Holmes comes to Seattle for his residency after three years in the Navy.

Petersdorf begins editing *Harrison's Principles of Internal Medicine*.

1968   Turck becomes chief of medicine at US Public Health Service Hospital.

Beaty becomes chief of infectious diseases at Harborview.

Holmes becomes Turck's first chief resident.

George Counts trains as ID fellow with Beaty.

1969   H. Hunter Handsfield begins internship, residency at UW.

1970–
1972   Paul Wiesner is King's first fellow.

1971   Petersdorf spends sabbatical at Beeson's Oxford laboratory, working on endocarditis.

1971–
1973   Handsfield trains as ID fellow with Holmes.

Walt Stamm does residency at UW.

1972   Jim Harnisch comes to the Seattle–King County Public Health Department as a CDC Venereal Diseases Division officer and simultaneously trains as ID fellow with Holmes.

1972–
1974   Joel Meyers serves in CDC's EIS.

| 1972–1981 | Stanley Falkow, who will mentor ID fellows, is professor of microbiology at UW. |

1972– Stanley Falkow, who will mentor ID fellows, is professor of
1981   microbiology at UW.

1973– David Eschenbach trains as ID fellow with Holmes.
1974

1973– Larry Corey serves in EIS.
1975

1973– Stamm serves in EIS, rising to branch chief.
1976

1974   EIS sends Meyers to Seattle to investigate an outbreak among bone marrow transplant patients.

American Medical Association establishes board certification for infectious diseases; Handsfield is in the first group to take the exam.

1974– Paul Beeson is distinguished Veterans Administration
1981   professor.

1975– Counts is ID chief at Harborview.
1984

1975   David Martin is chief resident at Public Health Service Hospital.

Lucy Tompkins arrives at Harborview for 3rd year of residency.

1975– Meyers is an ID fellow, though mostly works with E. Donnall
1976   Thomas.

1975– Corey trains as ID fellow with Holmes.
1977

1976– Klebanoff takes over from Kirby as head of newly combined
1994   and renamed UW Division of Allergy and Infectious Diseases.

1976– Stamm returns to Seattle to be chief resident at Harborview.
1977

1976– Martin trains as an ID fellow with Holmes.
1979

Tompkins trains as an ID fellow with Turck and Counts, then as a microbiology fellow with Stanley Falkow.

1977   Stamm trains as an ID fellow with Turck and Holmes.

Corey opens lab at Children's Hospital.

Meyers opens lab at Fred Hutch.

Kirby receives the Bristol Award from IDSA.

1978– 2005	Handsfield returns to Seattle after serving in the Navy to head the Sexually Transmitted Disease Control Program for Public Health Seattle—King County.
1978	Paul G. Ramsey arrives in Seattle as an ID fellow.
	Robert Brunham trains as an ID fellow with Holmes.
	Peter Piot trains as an ID fellow with Holmes.
1979	Sheila Lukehart trains as an ID fellow with Holmes.
	Tom Quinn trains as an ID fellow with Holmes.
	Edward W. Hook III, after completing his UW residency, serves as chief resident under Turck.
	Petersdorf leaves the UW to be president of Brigham and Women's Hospital, then vice chancellor for health sciences and dean of the School of Medicine at the University of California, San Diego.
1980	Ronald founds unit in Kenya for studying STDs with University of Nairobi.
1980– 1983	Hook trains as an ID fellow under Holmes.
1981	Harnisch opens a Seattle clinic to treat Hansen's disease, or leprosy.
	The CDC reports the first cases of what would later be named HIV/AIDS.
1980– 1983	Working with Trudy Elion, Corey demonstrates the effectiveness of acyclovir, the world's first antiviral therapy, for the treatment of herpes.
1982– 1984	Judith Wasserheit trains as an ID fellow with Holmes and David Eschenbach.
1982– 1985	Ann Collier trains as an ID fellow with Hunter Handsfield.
1982– 1986	Anne Rompalo trains as an ID fellow.
1984	Holmes's fellow Joan Kreiss joins Ronald to study AIDS in Kenyan female sex workers.
1985	Collier and Kreiss found Madison Clinic, which Collier directs until 1990.
1986	Bob Wood becomes medical director of Seattle–King County AIDS Control Program.

1986   Sherris retires.

1986–   Wesley Van Voorhis trains as an ID fellow with Klebanoff.
1989

1987–   Larry Corey organizes and oversees AIDS Clinical Trials Group.
1992

1988   Holmes and Kreiss form the UW International AIDS Research and Training Program.

1989–   Connie Celum trains as an ID fellow with Holmes.
1991

1989–   Turck is editor of *The Journal of Infectious Diseases*
2002

1990–   Ramsey is UW chair of medicine.
1997

1991   Meyers dies of colon cancer; landmark paper on ganciclovir and CMV published posthumously.

1991–   Anna Wald trains as an ID fellow with Larry Corey.
1994

1992–   Jeanne Marrazzo trains as an ID fellow with Hunter Handsfield.
1994

1993   Klebanoff wins Bristol Award from IDSA.

1994–   Stamm is head of ID division.
2007

1995   Petersdorf retires as president of Association of American Medical Colleges and returns to UW as adviser at VA Medical Center and to dean of medical school.

1996   Corey moves to Fred Hutch to head its Vaccine and Infectious Disease Division.

1997   Kirby dies at 82.

1999   Corey organizes HIV Vaccine Trials Network.

2002   Eschenbach named chair of UW Department of Obstetrics and Gynecology.

2005   Stamm serves as president of IDSA.

2006   Holmes becomes founding chair of UW Department of Global Health.

Beeson dies at 97.

Petersdorf dies at 80.

2007   Klebanoff receives Association of American Medical Colleges' lifetime research award.

2007– Van Voorhis heads ID Division.
2017

2009   Stamm dies at 64.

2013   Holmes wins IDSA Bristol award (now Alexander Fleming Award).

2014   Wasserheit succeeds Holmes as chair of UW Global Health.

2016   Klebanoff dies at 87.

2017   Anna Wald becomes head of UW ID division.

2021   John Sherris dies at 100.

MAJOR AWARDS

Infectious Diseases Society of America Alexander Fleming Award (formerly the Bristol Award), for lifetime achievement

Paul Beeson (1972)
Bill Kirby (1977)
Seymour Klebanoff (1993)
King Holmes (2013)

Bristol-Myers Squibb Award for Distinguished Achievement in Infectious Disease Research

Seymour Klebanoff (1995)

Gairdner Foundation Awards

Allan Ronald (Wightman Award, 2006)
King Holmes (Global Health Award, 2013)
Peter Piot (Global Health Award, 2015)

American Sexually Transmitted Diseases Association (ASTDA) Distinguished Career Award

King K. Holmes (1983)
E. Russell Alexander (1984)
Paul Wiesner (1989)
Allan Ronald (1991)
Lawrence Corey (1997)
Peter Piot (1998)
Robert B. Jones (1999)
Walter E. Stamm (2000)
Robert C. Brunham (2004)
Sheila A. Lukehart (2007)
Edward W. Hook III (2008)
Sharon Hillier (2009)
H. Hunter Handsfield (2010)
Thomas C. Quinn (2011)
David Martin (2012)
Anna Wald (2015)
Anne Marie Rompalo (2016)

ASTDA Achievement Award recognizing an outstanding body of work or a single major achievement at midcareer

Paul Wiesner (1975)
Lawrence Corey (1984)
Sheila A. Lukehart (1991)
Walter E. Stamm (1995)
Sharon Hillier (1996)
Judith N. Wasserheit (1997)
Thomas C. Quinn (1999)
Edward W. Hook III (2000)
Anna Wald (2004)
David Martin (2006)
Connie Celum (2011)
Kim Workowski (2012)
Jane Schwebke (2013)
Christina Marra (2014)
Jeanne Marrazzo (2015)

Acknowledgments

I'm profoundly grateful for the researchers and clinicians who allowed me to tell their stories in *Hot Spot*.

Larry Corey and King Holmes were especially generous and supportive in thinking through this project and reviewing it, while at the same time trusting me to tell the story ("Off you go!") without interference. H. Hunter Handsfield helped enormously with ideas and feedback and contributed many photos from his personal collection (the blackmail-worthy ones he is holding on to), as did King.

Robert Brunham, Helen Chu, Ann Collier, George Counts, David Eschenbach, James Harnisch, Ned Hook, Sheila Lukehart, Jeanne Marrazzo, David Martin, Patricia McInturff, Peter Piot, Tom Quinn, Allan Ronald, the late John Sherris, Lucy Tompkins, Marvin Turck, Wes Van Voorhis, Anna Wald, Judy Wasserheit, and Bob Wood shared memories not just of their own experiences but of their mentors, trainees, and colleagues. They did so with enthusiasm for the science, compassion for their patients, and humor about themselves.

Barbara Kirby and Richard Kirby told wonderful stories of their late father, William Kirby, and made me wish I'd had a chance to meet him. The late Donald Kaye, an infectious-diseases pioneer in his own right, lent a valuable perspective from outside Seattle. Many others in Seattle's ID community shared insights with me that in one way or another found their way into this book, including Trevor Bedford,

Michael Boeckh, Keith Jerome, Rhoda Ashley Morrow, Steve Pergam, and Steve Wakefield.

Beth Minnich, executive assistant to Larry Corey, and Elisabeth Gunningham, executive assistant to King Holmes, helped immeasurably by carving time for interviews out of insanely busy schedules, finding documents, tracking down decades-old photos, and so much more. Aleta Elliott, executive assistant to Judy Wallerstein, also deserves special thanks. Eric Chow somehow found time during his own ID fellowship to assemble a list of past fellows, which he kindly shared with me along with other research documents.

Additional help finding photos came from Kim Blakely of UW School of Medicine communications and Rachel Cascio of Fred Hutchinson Cancer Research Center's Arnold Library. Thanks also to those who gave permission for the use of photographs, including *The Seattle Times*, the Association of American Medical Colleges, and the American Federation for Aging Research. Photographer and friend Robert Hood generously volunteered his time to fine-tune dozens of images.

Editor Cindy Jensen's careful reading and corrections improved the book immensely. Thank you to Bryan Tomasovich of The Publishing World for the clear and distinctive interior design and for overseeing and managing the publishing process, and Patrick Grandaw for his evocative cover design. I'm also grateful to Siri Carpenter and Luke Timmerman for the time they took to walk me through all they'd learned about publishing from their own books.

I am indebted to the authors whose books were an invaluable resource for this project, especially *Fulfilling the Dream: A History of the University of Washington School of Medicine, 1946 to 1988* by Clement A. Finch, *No Time to Lose: A Life in Pursuit of Deadly Viruses* by Peter Piot, and *Physician: The Life of Paul Beeson* by Richard Rapport.

Excellent reporting by Sheri Fink and Mike Baker in *The New York Times*; Shawn Boburg, Robert O'Harrow Jr., Neena Satija, and Amy Goldstein in *The Washington Post*; and Alice Park in *Time* magazine helped me re-create Seattle's role in the early days of the COVID-19 pandemic. Both the National Institutes of Health and the Seattle-King County Department of Public Health maintain oral history archives of the AIDS pandemic, including interviews with several of the people featured in this history, which were both helpful and extraordinarily moving. I first met some of the scientists featured in this history when

I worked as a writer for Fred Hutchinson Cancer Research Center's news service; my work there and that of my talented colleagues helped inform this book.

I am lucky and thankful to have in my husband Nolan Hester both a supportive cheerleader—especially needed when this book took longer than expected—and a keen-eyed editor.

I also appreciate the continued enthusiasm for this project (and the patience) of all those I interviewed. About the time I thought I would have this book wrapped up, COVID-19 happened. Talk about a reminder of why infectious-diseases research matters. Seattle researchers and the generations they've trained and are training were in the thick of it. For that, we can all be grateful.

Index

(Page numbers in *italics* refer to illustrations.)

A

Index

D

Dale, David C., 56

Dalkon shield, 52

Dartmouth College, 69, 109, 110–11

Davis, Gray, 145

Democratic Republic of Congo, 84, 120, 155

dendritic cells, 136

dermatology, ix, xii, 45, 53, 106, 129–31

Diaz, George, 157

diphtheria, 2, 53–55, 83

disseminated gonococcal infection (DGI), ix, 43

doctor draft, 27, 42, 45, 77

Dowdle, Walter, 59

Dowling, Harry F., 15

Duchin, Jeffrey, 162

E

Ebola, 84–85, 150, 155, 157, 159, 162

EIS, *see* Epidemic Intelligence Service

Elion, Gertrude, 64–65, 145, 186

Emory University School of Medicine, 3, 4, 45, 132

endocarditis, v, 54–55, 61, 72, 80

Englund, Janet, 158

Epidemic Intelligence Service, vi, ix, x, 14–16, 45, 56–60, 62, 63, 71, 72, 85, 123–24, 150, 183, 184, 185

Eschenbach, David A., ix, xi, *99, 101,* 115, 123, 133–134, 150, 187, 190

    early years, 49-55, 71–72, 185

Evans, Charles, 11

F

Falkow, Stanley, 61–62, 69–71, 82, 85, 185

Fauci, Anthony, 115, 117, 135, 148, 154, 163

FDA (Food and Drug Administration), 21, 161, 164

"Fever of Unexplained Origin," 5, 183

Fielder, Mary, 151

Finland, Maxwell, 8, 15, 62, 166

Florey, Mary Ethel, 10

flu, *see* influenza

Folsome, Clair E., 28

Francis, Tommy, 57–59

Fred Hutchinson Cancer Research Center (Fred Hutch), xii, 66, 73, 115, 119, 123–29, 137, 148–49, 154, 157–161, 164, 185, 187, 191, 192

Fredricks, David, xi, 144

G

Gairdner Awards, 188

Galloway, Denise, 137

ganciclovir, 124–125, 187

gay and bisexual men, *see also* men who have sex with men, 47–49, 87–88, 91, 106–14, 142

gay rights, 47, 88, 117, 121, 141

global health, vii, x, xi, 121, 132, 135, 147, 158, 165, 187, 188

Global Health, UW Department of, vii, xi, 135, 147, 187

gonorrhea, ix, 29–30, 38, 39–40, 43, 46–47, 49–50, 63, 69, 75–80, 82, 198, 118, 134, 144

Index

149, 151-52, 154, 188, 189, 190

   early years, 109, 123, 132–35, 140, 186

Wear, Jennifer, 47

Weill Cornell Medical College, vi, 6, 7, 26, 70, 80, 136

Weiss, Soma, 3

West Coast vs. East Coast, xii–xiii, 67, 70

Western blot test, 85, 146

WHO (World Health Organization), 86, 156

Wiesner, Paul, vii–ix, 37–39, 42–44, 47, 49, 51–53, 63, *105*, 184, 189

Williams, Robert H., 7, 9, 16, 18, 33

Wilson, Chris, 89, 137

Winter, Carol, 64–65

women in infectious diseases field, x–xi, 69, 71, 74–76, 140–44, 153

Wood, Robert "Bob," *100*, 110–14, 118, 121, 186, 190

Wood, W. Barry, 6, 166, 170n24

Woodward, Theodore E., 23, 166

World War II, 1, 8, 10, 29, 39, 57, 61, 166

Worth, Robert, 28, 130

Y

Yale School of Medicine, v, 1–4, 6, 13, 19, 54, 94, 143, 166

Z

Zaire *see also* Democratic Republic of Congo, 84–85, 120

Zika virus, 155, 159

Mary Engel is an award-winning healthcare writer who has worked for newspapers in California, Alaska, and New Mexico and as a science writer for the Fred Hutchinson Cancer Research Center. The editorials she wrote for the *Los Angeles Times* were part of a 2005 Pulitzer Prize-winning series on mismanagement, malpractice, and racial injustice at a public hospital. She has been a Knight Science Journalism Fellow at MIT, a science journalism fellow at the Marine Biological Laboratory in Woods Hole, Mass., and a Salzburg Seminar Knight Media Fellow on multicultural healthcare in Salzburg, Austria. She lives in Seattle.

CPSIA information can be obtained
at www.ICGtesting.com
Printed in the USA
JSHW051705120822
29198JS00001B/3